The Woman's Guide to Strength Training
Dumbbells

Women's Health

The Woman's Guide to Strength Training
Dumbbells

Nellie Barnett, CPT,
and the editors of *Women's Health*

Table of Contents

Introduction: Your Strongest Era Starts Now 7

Strength Training Basics 8

How the Plan Works 18

Your 12-Week Dumbbell Strength-Training Plan 24

- **Prep Stage**
  - Week 1 27
  - Week 2 28

- **Stage 1**
  - Week 1 30
  - Week 2 38
  - Week 3 46
  - Week 4 54

- **Stage 2**
  - Week 5 63
  - Week 6 72
  - Week 7 82
  - Week 8 92

- **Stage 3**
  - Week 9 103
  - Week 10 112
  - Week 11 122
  - Week 12 132

Dumbbell Exercise Glossary 144

Upper Body

Cat Cow	144
I-Y-T Raise	145
Thread the Needle	146
Pushup	147
Cross-Body Alternating Biceps Curl	148
Hammer Curl	149
Wide Biceps Curl	150
Zottman Curl	151
Overhead Triceps Extension	152
Chest Fly	153
Reverse Fly	154
Alternating Reverse Fly	155
Halo	156
Arnold Press	157
Bridge Chest Press	158
Chest Press	159
Alternating Chest Press	160
Gator Press	161
Dumbbell Seesaw Press	162
Shoulder Press	163
Kneeling Dumbbell Shoulder Press	164
Single-Arm Shoulder Press	165
Lateral Raise	166
Alternating Front and Lateral Raise	167
Dumbbell Rainbow	168
Alternating Bent-Over Row	169
Gorilla Row	170
Dumbbell Single-Arm Row	171
Underhand Bent-Over Row	172
Upright Row	173
Skull Crusher	174

Core

Side Plank Hip Dip	175
Deadbug	176
Loaded Deadbug	177
Russian Twist	178
Weighted Russian Twist	179
Toe Touch	180
Wood Chop	181

Lower Body

High Knee	182
Glute Bridge	183
Romanian Deadlift	184
Staggered-Stance Deadlift	185
Weighted Hip Thrust	186
Deficit Reverse Lunge	187
Lateral Lunge	188
Two-Way Lunge	189
Squat	190
Back Squat	191
Bulgarian Split Squat	192
Goblet Squat	193
Front Racked Squat	194
Staggered-Stance Front Racked Squat	195
Dumbbell Sumo Squat	196
Squat Jump	197
Dumbbell Swing	198

Total Body

World's Greatest Stretch	199
Plank Walkout	200
Modified Burpee	201
Reverse Lunge to Press	202
Modified Devil Press	203
Dumbbell Speed Skater	204
Squat and Snatch	205
Squat Thruster	206

introduction

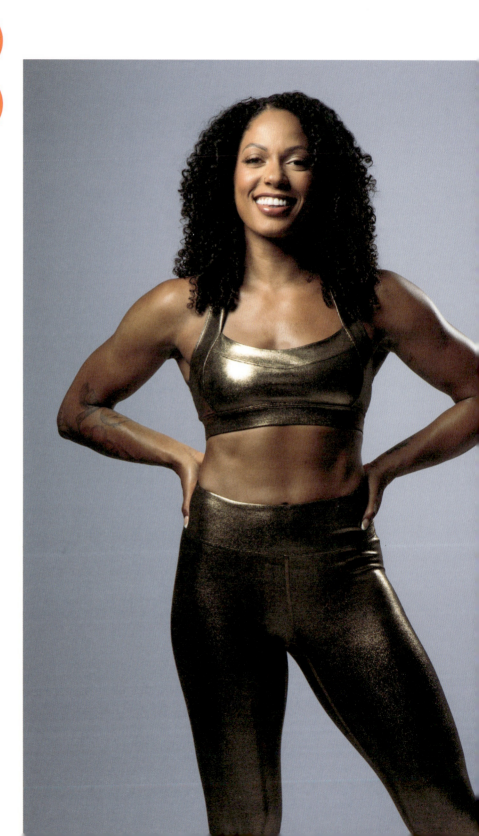

Your Strongest Era Starts Now

What if I told you strength training will change your life—and nearly every part of it? Not just how much weight you can lift or the size of your muscles, but the way you approach any challenge that comes your way? That's how it changed mine.

I'm Nellie Barnett, CPT, a fitness and wellness coach who empowers women to unlock their full potential with activities focused on the body, mind, and soul through my business, Nellbells Fitness. Before I was deadlifting barbells and swinging kettlebells (and loving it!), I didn't always prioritize physical activity. I ate relatively healthy, but I wasn't consistently active. I'd hit the gym for one week and then stop going for two months, try a bootcamp class or run a few times a week but then eventually fall back into old habits. Sound familiar? Nothing seemed to keep my interest, and I'd always find a reason not to keep up with my workouts.

Year after year my goal was "get toned," and year after year it didn't happen. That is, until something shifted in me. I could credit it to prioritizing my health, but it was much deeper than that. I felt like life was happening to me, but I was ready to make life happen for me.

So I started working out consistently and introducing new dumbbell and barbell workouts into my fitness routine. I was amazed by the versatility of dumbbells. The physical benefits were great—toned arms, feeling stronger, more energy—but it was the mental boost that kept me coming back. This epiphany awakened my inner willpower, and from that moment on, strength training became my salvation.

I stayed true to my goals both in and out of the gym (like working out Monday through Friday and finally booking that solo trip I'd always dreamed of) to prove to myself that I am worthy and capable of all that I desire.

When I first entered the gym, I didn't even know what a burpee was. I never would have imagined that I would be deadlifting one day…let alone 285 pounds! Over time, I developed a growth mindset in all areas of life. You will shatter your own expectations, too, when you start strength training. With this program, you can build the strength and mental resilience that'll make every day easier—and you can do it all from home with just a set of dumbbells. You don't need expensive gym equipment, bulky barbells, or even a full rack of weights to build strong arms, legs, abs, and the unstoppable mindset that comes with it. You just need to follow the plan in this book.

My strategic 12-week strength-training program will show you how to get the most out of a few dumbbells using powerful exercises, muscle-boosting techniques, and workouts that build on one another. It features the principles I've seen work for myself and my clients again and again. If you're a beginner, dumbbells offer a low-cost and uncomplicated entrance to the world of strength training. And if you're already familiar with this tool, you know how versatile it can be. Dumbbells don't take up much room in your home, and you can do a lot with just one set.

If you're ready to unlock boundless strength, build muscle all over, and cultivate willpower like never before, you're in the right place. Whether you're starting your own fitness journey or just want to switch up your workouts, you'll find a manageable and effective path in this program.

Before we dive in, let's go over some basics that will set you up for success. —*Nellie Barnett, CPT*

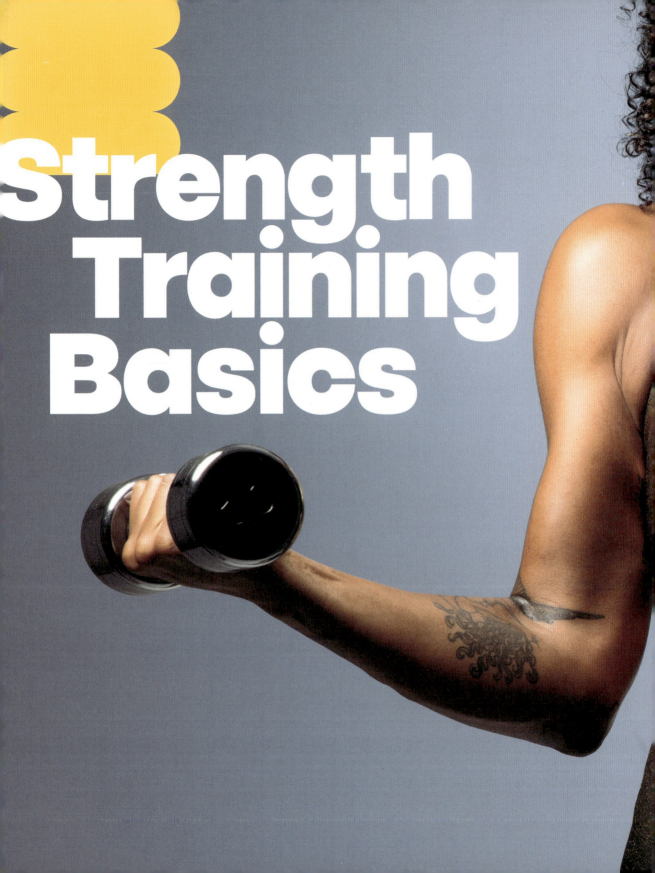

Strength Training Basics

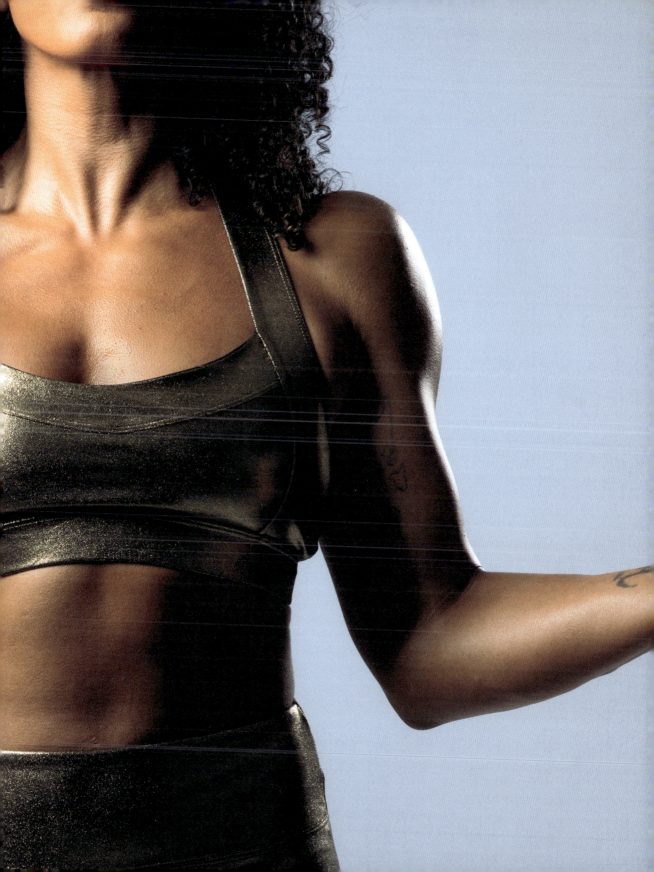

Strength Training Basics

YOU MIGHT ENVISION stacks of weight plates and barbells when you think of strength training, but building muscle doesn't have to be that complicated. Simply put, strength training (a.k.a. resistance training) involves using either your own body weight or equipment—like dumbbells or resistance bands—to build muscle mass, strength, and endurance.

Exactly what results you get depends on your starting point, the resistance you use, the type of training you do, plus other factors. One thing's for sure: Whether you're getting creative with bodyweight exercises or moving heavy weights at the gym, it'll help you build muscle, boost your metabolism, and improve your overall health. Here's what else you should know about strength training before getting started.

It's Good for More Than Your Muscles

Defined arms and strong abs are just the beginning of the long list of benefits you'll get to experience when you incorporate strength training into your fitness journey. When you start to see physical results and then notice improvements in your mental health, your self-image will start to shift in the most empowering way. These results typically take only weeks to notice and include defined muscles, more energy, and revved up metabolism. Strength training can also help you:

Build stronger bones and joints

Resistance exercises not only help grow muscle mass but also put stress on your bones, which stimulates bone growth and increases bone density. Stronger, denser bones equals greater protection against injury and can contribute to reducing the risk of osteoporosis and fractures later in life. You'll also strengthen and protect your joints with movements that loosen those stiff and achy areas.

Improve stabilization

Everything you do on your feet—from hustling

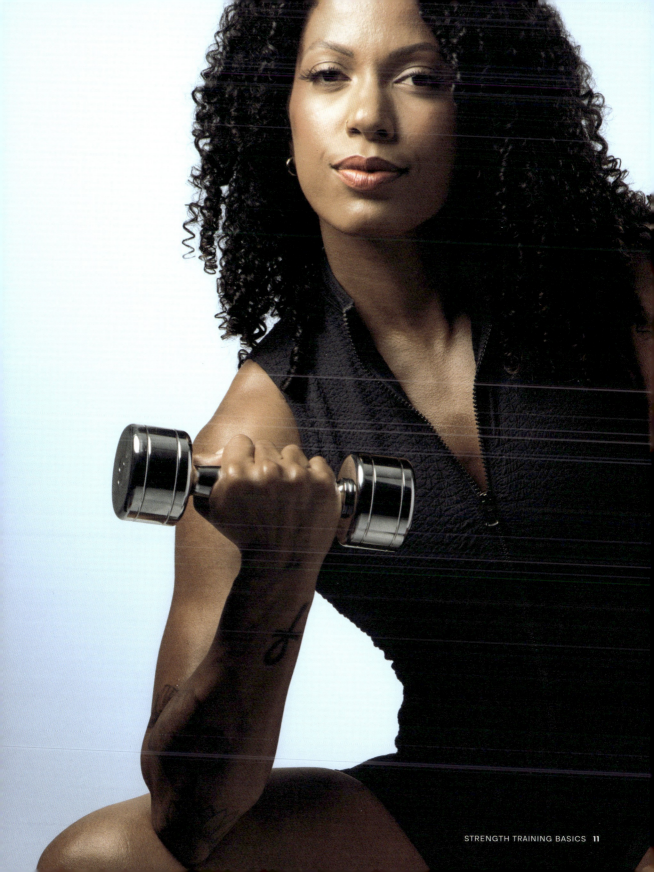

Strength Training Basics

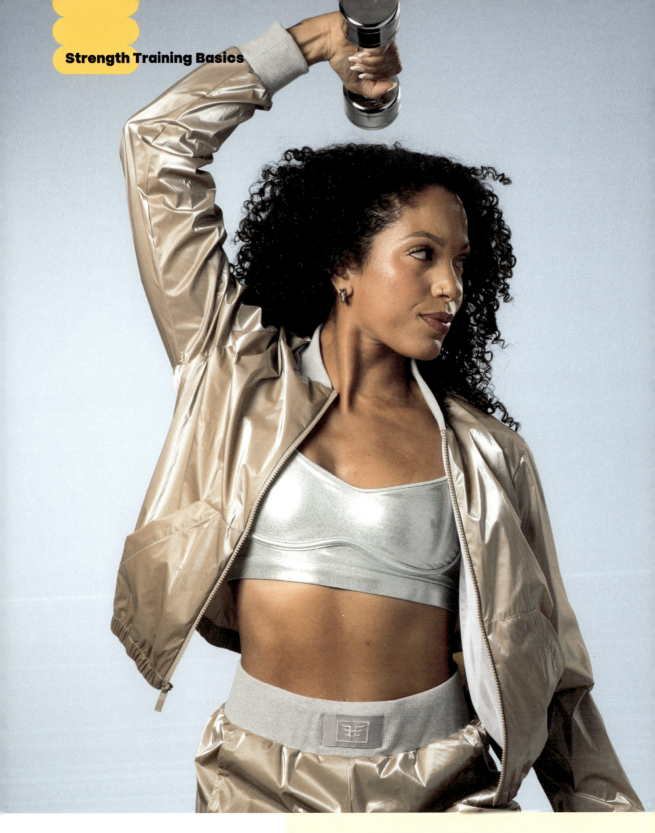

up the stairs to taking a stroll around the block—requires stability. Without it, you'd wobble through your daily to-dos. All resistance training strengthens your stabilizer muscles, which are responsible for keeping you steady, but dumbbell exercises are especially effective. They require your body to counter the weight you're holding, especially when performing single arm or single leg movements, since this engages your core and stabilizer muscles more. With a foundation of strong stabilizer muscles you'll lower your risk of injury—particularly during exercise, when misalignment, poor balance, and improper form can often cause you to tweak a muscle.

Boost body image

You might notice a surge of body positivity after hitting the weights—and there's research to prove it. Several studies have looked at the relationship between body image and strength training and found that women report more positive feelings about their bodies after completing resistance-training programs compared to those who don't. In a study published in the *American Journal of Health Promotion*, that was the case for the 62 women who reported more positive body images after lifting weights twice per week for 15 weeks compared to 92 women in the study who didn't strength train.

Do everyday activities with less stress

Getting stronger just makes daily life easier. Think: carrying groceries from your car in one trip and having tons of energy to keep up with pets or little ones while playing. Plus, the improved balance, coordination, and flexibility you'll experience will make all types of activities feel easier and smoother. Strength training often includes compound exercises—moves that use multiple muscle groups—which mimic and help you prepare for movements you regularly do in real life. For example, the proper form and technique you learn over time from doing deadlifts is going to make picking up heavy boxes or moving furniture a breeze. That's because deadlifts engage the hamstrings, glutes, lower back, and core. One more bonus: Strength training boosts your mental health, giving you the confidence to tackle anything life throws your way.

Increase calorie burn and decrease body fat

If weight loss is your goal, strength training can certainly help increase your calorie burn. When consistently paired with proper nutrition, it can result in muscle-mass increase and a higher resting metabolic rate (the amount of calories your body burns at rest).

Another cool side effect: As your body is recovering from a strength workout, it experiences excess post-exercise oxygen consumption (EPOC), which basically means your body is consuming more oxygen and burning more calories than usual for up to several hours after a sweat session.

Step up your cardiovascular health

More and more studies show that strength training can improve heart health just as effectively as cardio. After looking at data from more than 400,000 people as part of a two-decades-long analysis, research from the *Journal of the American College of Cardiology* in 2024 found that women who strength trained had a 30 percent reduced risk of cardiovascular-related death.

Additionally, the results of a 2019 study published in *Medicine & Science in Sports & Exercise* found that people who did at least one hour of strength training per week had a 40 to 70 percent lower risk of heart attack or stroke compared to those who didn't.

Alleviate depression symptoms

You already know exercise can be a major mood lifter, but did you know resistance training in particular can have feel-good effects? A meta-analysis published in *JAMA Psychiatry* looked at 33 studies (a total of almost 1,900 subjects between them) to see if resistance training had any sizable positive impact on easing depressive symptoms. It determined that not only does strength training boost physical strength, but it also improves low mood, loss of interest in activities, and feelings of worthlessness, showing how interconnected our mind and body are.

Strength Training Basics

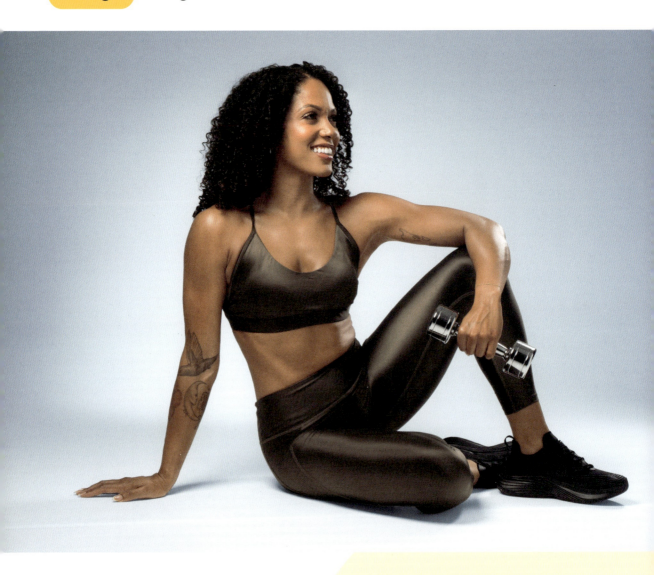

Your Fitness Goals, Unlocked

Most people tend to think of strength training as simply lifting weights or using resistance to build muscle, but there's more to it than just "picking things up and putting them down." Varying different elements, like your rest time between sets or total rep count, can help you target and smash specific goals, whether you want to build stamina, strength, or size.

IF YOU WANT TO: Sculpt muscle and build strength
TRY: Hypertrophy training

This is what we'll primarily focus on in the 12-week plan. Hypertrophy training increases the size of your muscles using exercises performed with medium to heavy weight (usually 6–12 repetitions for 3–6 sets). Your muscle fibers tear during the workout and then grow and get stronger during your rest days. That's usually why hypertrophy training schedules include workouts that focus on one muscle group at a time, so your upper body gets a chance to rest when leg day rolls around. This is a popular form of training to build a sculpted physique.

**IF YOU WANT TO: Build stamina and resilience
TRY: Muscle endurance training**

This approach involves higher repetitions (usually 12 or more) and lighter weights, while focusing on sustaining the same level of effort. This is a great approach for beginners because it will build up your muscle tissues in order to progress to more challenging workouts. It's also commonly used by endurance athletes for sports like running, cycling, etc., and it's great for boosting your overall daily energy. We'll weave in some muscle endurance training in the optional 2-week prep stage of the plan, which I strongly recommend.

**IF YOU WANT TO: Combine your cardio and strength training
TRY: Circuit training**

You don't have to give up cardio to hit your strength goals. Circuit training actually combines the best of both worlds, giving you a cardiovascular workout while improving muscle strength and endurance. You'll get your heart rate up by performing a series of exercises consecutively with minimal rest between sets. Circuit workouts are made up of multiple exercises that usually target multiple muscle groups, with the goal of completing one full circuit and then repeating it for multiple rounds.

**IF YOU WANT TO: Lift really heavy objects
TRY: Max strength training**

There's no feeling quite like being able to easily lift something extremely heavy. Max strength training can make that happen. It's all about tapping into your body's full strength potential and pushing past any limits. It's like cranking the intensity dial all the way up by using heavy weights and doing low repetitions (no more than 6). This allows you to lift the heaviest weight possible for compound movements such as squats, bench presses, and deadlifts. This type of training develops brute force for maximal strength gains.

**IF YOU WANT TO: Lift really heavy objects quickly
TRY: Explosive power training**

If you want to move heavy things fast, you'll need some of this in your routine. Explosive power training is an advanced training style where strength is exerted as quickly as possible in a given exercise, typically for 1–2 repetitions. A great example of this is Olympic power lifting because the snatch and clean and jerk are movements that require explosive strength and force.

As you can see, there are plenty of different ways to reap the benefits of strength training and this 12-week program is the perfect place to start! I created this plan to help you build muscle, get stronger, and boost your endurance with one simple program. Whether you're a beginner or you've incorporated strength training into your normal fitness routine, this book will help you keep your body strong and healthy.

Dumbbells Are Just as Powerful as the Gym

You can get incredible results with weight machines and barbells, but all the gear in the world won't matter if you never find time to use it. Dumbbells solve the time crunch by saving you a commute to the gym. They're small enough to stash under your bed and can be used even in the most compact apartments. When your gym is at home, you'll be even more likely to follow through on a routine. Plus, the fact that dumbbells are one of the most budget-friendly and widely available tools on the market makes it that much easier to get one step closer to your strength goals.

Aside from being convenient and affordable, dumbbells also pack a lot of power into a small package. When used strategically, they can strengthen all the same muscles as a roomful of equipment. Plus, unlike weight machines, which often isolate a single muscle, dumbbells allow you to move in a wider range of motion while isolating a single muscle or incorporating movements that simultaneously work various body parts.

Selecting the right weight for your fitness level and goals is key. As you now know, your end goal–

Strength Training Basics

whether it's to build muscle or boost endurance—will determine which of the previously mentioned strength-training modalities you should follow and the weight range you should use. For example, if you're doing explosive power training, you'll want to use heavy weights for just a few reps. If you're following a hypertrophy training plan, you'll use medium to heavy weights. But what's heavy to one person may feel light to another. So how do you find the correct weight for you? Here are some simple rules to follow:

Find the Right Weight for You

For beginners: You shouldn't go from zero to bench-pressing 150 pounds (I know you know this). If you're trying out a new exercise or workout, start with just your body weight! It may sound simple, but mastering proper form and technique is essential for injury prevention. Once you have the form down, lighter weights will become your best friends. The key is mastering the technique and learning to engage your muscles with mind-muscle connection—you'll learn more about that soon. Gradually you can either up your reps or increase the weight for more of a challenge.

When you're ready to lift heavier: The best advice to follow is to start with a weight that feels manageable to you without compromising your form. A great test for what's considered "manageable" is whether or not you're able to complete the repetitions with good form and feel challenged toward the end of each set. For example, when performing 10 reps, if you are struggling by rep 3 and your form is getting sloppy, then that's a good indication that you need to go down in weight. When you're able to get through all reps with good form, while still feeling challenged with the last few reps, that's when you've found your sweet spot. The last 3 reps of your set should be hard, while maintaining proper form, whether that's a total rep count of 20 (light weight), 12 (medium weight), or 6 (heavy weight). From there you can gradually increase the weight over time to allow your muscles time to adapt to the new weight.

Considerations: You'll find that the amount of weight you're able to curl is dramatically different from the amount you're able to squat, and that's because different muscle groups have varying capacities for lifting weights due to the size of the muscle, the muscle fibers, the mechanics involved for a particular movement, and whether it's a compound movement. If you're unsure of what weight to use, start lighter and do the rep test mentioned above.

Once you've mastered proper form and mind-muscle connection, consistency is what matters when it comes to getting the full benefit of dumbbells. Aim to lift challenging weights three to five times per week and mix in some active recovery like we do in this program. Doing so keeps your muscles and frame strong and mobile, plus it's manageable to stick with long term. Research shows that bone mass peaks for most women in their late 20s, and density starts to dwindle in their early 40s. So finding a strength-training program you can follow throughout your life will help support you in the long run.

4 Essential Elements of an Effective Strength-Training Routine

Crafting a workout regimen that is sustainable, efficient, and fun is key to consistency in your fitness journey. And when you're consistent, you're more likely to reach your goal in no time. Here are four key pieces you should have in any strength routine you try.

1. A Firm Schedule

You probably wouldn't think of skipping your next doctor's appointment, right? So treat your training the same way by picking a time and day to work out and note it in your calendar. One of the hardest parts about being consistent is creating a routine that you will stick to! Personally, I like to work out in the early morning so nothing gets in the way, and it starts my day off right. Test different workout times until you find your perfect fit. The workouts in this program should take approximately 30–45 minutes and can be done at home, so they're perfect for adding to your a.m. routine.

2. An Effective (and Fun!) Warm-up

You'll be more likely to adhere to your workout if you feel good doing it, and taking a few minutes to warm up your muscles is one of the best ways to ensure you hit the weights feeling great. Wake your body up with dynamic stretches, which use gentle movement to limber up your muscles and get your blood flowing. Take this time to notice any tightness in your muscles or discomfort you may feel in your body; those are the areas that need some extra TLC. Getting your body warmed up for the workout is also key to aid in injury prevention. This program includes a quick warm-up to get you primed and ready for each workout!

3. Lots of Variety

Switching your workout up doesn't just keep you from getting bored, it also boosts your results. Following this 12-week program is a great way to try a new regimen and learn about strength-training techniques, and my hope is that when you finish, you continue your strength journey. As you create your own workouts, make sure to modify your training variables (as you will in this program) such as intensity, volume, frequency, and exercise selection to continue challenging your body and stimulating muscle growth. When you plan out your workouts for the week, include different movements such as push (e.g., chest press), pull (e.g., dumbbell row), squats, lunges, and hinge movements. When performing these movements, gradually increase the weight lifted, perform different movement patterns, vary the number of sets and repetitions, and introduce new exercises or training techniques to keep workouts fresh and engaging.

4. A Holistic Recovery Strategy

Strength training is hard work, so you have to devote as much attention to recovering from your training as you do to your time at the weights. After all, you can't operate on empty! To ensure you enter your next workout feeling energized and at optimal health, focus on getting enough sleep, eating nutritious foods, staying hydrated, managing stress, and doing active recovery (any physical activity that's low intensity). See the tips at right for easy ways to boost your recovery.

How to Feel Your Best Every. Single. Workout.

What you do while away from the weights can mean the difference between breezing through your reps and dragging from move to move. Follow these tips to start every workout on the right foot.

Hydrate Fully
Weigh yourself then divide that number by two to figure out how many ounces of water you should drink per day.

Minimize Stress
Try self-care activities like slathering on a relaxing face mask or meditating for a few minutes to help you unwind.

Sleep Soundly
Skip caffeine later in the day, avoid looking at screens before bed, and keep your bedroom completely dark to encourage deep Zs.

Keep Moving
One active recovery day per week is one of the best ways to alleviate muscle soreness! Try going on long walks, stretching, foam rolling, doing yoga—anything that gently moves your body.

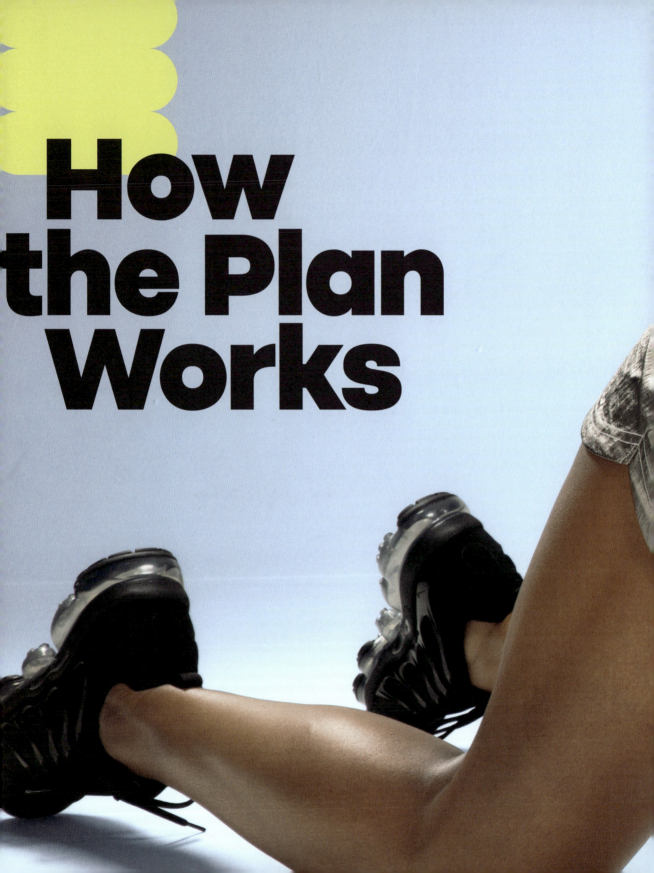
How the Plan Works

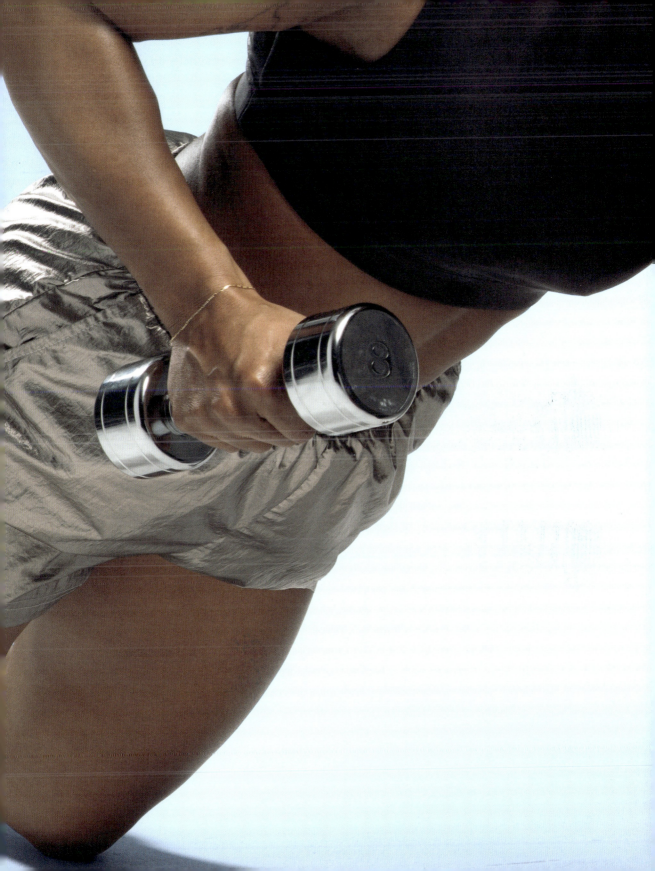

How the Plan Works

Are you ready to get stronger, sculpt your muscles, and feel empowered from the comfort of your own home?

Before you pick up the weights, here's what to expect over the next 12 weeks.

This program is designed for all fitness levels. Whether you're new to this or experienced, we're bringing the gym to you, using nothing but dumbbells and your determination. This 12-week program is divided into three stages with an optional 2-week prep stage. Each stage builds on the work you did in the stage before it and amps up the intensity just enough to increase your gains without overwhelming you. This strategy, known as progressive overload, gradually dials up the challenge on your muscles—either through more frequent workouts, heavier weights, or higher reps, etc. In this plan, you'll use all three, boosting your results without wearing yourself out.

You'll work out three to four times per week for about 30–45 minutes per workout. What time of day you work out is up to you, but I find scheduling it for a predetermined time increases the chance that life won't get in the way of your fitness goals.

If you'd like to keep these workouts to 30 minutes, follow this:

1 Perform the three-minute warm up (shown above each daily workout chart) to get you ready for the workout.

2 Most of the workouts include four different exercises. Grab yourself a timer and set it for six minutes. During that time you will perform all of the sets of one exercise before moving to the next. The goal is to complete all three sets within the six minutes before moving to the next exercise.

3 When the timer goes off, you have one minute to get ready for the next exercise. Set your six-minute timer and get moving! Repeat until you complete all exercises.

While doing this program, I want you to show up fully for yourself—both during and outside of your workouts. Stay committed to getting the workouts done. For the ultimate results, you will need to eat colorful meals made up of veggies, fruits, complex carbohydrates, and protein. At a bare minimum, follow the American College of Sports Medicine's guideline of consuming at least 1.2 to 1.7 grams of protein per kilogram of body weight per day, or 0.5 to 0.8 grams per pound of body weight. You'll likely need to up your intake to fit your needs and goals, but a general benchmark of 20 to 30 grams of protein per meal will set you in the right direction.

What You'll Need

I've designed this plan to give you the most bang for your buck, so it doesn't require much.

▶ 3 Pairs of Dumbbells

Follow the guidelines for picking the right weight for you from page 16. To further boost results, consider getting a **light**, **medium**, and **heavy pair** so you can adjust the weight based on the exercise you're doing.

▶ 1 Yoga Mat

You'll get on the ground for some exercises, so a **cushy mat will make these moves more comfortable.**

Protein is essential because it provides the necessary amino acids that your body needs to repair and build muscle. Whenever you work out, and especially when you strength train, your muscle fibers are tearing at the microscopic level and then rebuilding with the help of sufficient amino acids. Protein also helps you feel fuller longer, so if you're a snacker, it'll help curb that tendency.

If this is all new to you then I want you to take it one step at a time and aim to have some form of protein with each meal (don't worry about the numbers). That can be eggs, fish, chicken, beans, etc. If you feel you are not getting enough protein in your regular diet, then you can incorporate supplements such as protein shakes and bars. By prioritizing protein and whole foods you are giving your body what it needs to build and maintain muscle.

How the Plan Works

> ## My Favorite Way to Do Active Recovery
>
> I like to go for long walks. Not only does it help me keep my muscles moving, it's also a way for me to take a mental health break. No screens; just the beautiful outdoors!

The Stages

Breaking your training into distinct phases will supercharge your results for a few reasons. For one, it makes the plan feel more manageable and establishes natural checkpoints for you to celebrate the work you've done and reflect on how far you've come. More importantly, it allows you to employ that progressive overload strategy mentioned earlier. In each stage of this plan, you'll vary your workload in some way to further challenge your muscles and trigger growth.

Each of the three stages lasts four weeks. That gives you just enough time to get comfortable with the movements and, by the final week of each stage, get ready to start ramping it up. Within each stage there are multiple workouts, active recovery days, and rest days. Active recovery encourages gentle movement to promote blood flow which will aid in reducing muscle soreness from those days when you're going hard. This can include walking, swimming, and stretching, just to name a few. For strong muscles, rest is just as important as the work you put in. Here's what you'll gain from each stage.

Optional Prep Stage: Proper Form

Strength-training beginner? Start here. If you're coming back after a break or already train regularly, this is still a great opportunity to recommit to perfect form. Either way, you'll lay a foundation to build upon, which will make tackling the full plan easier. The focus is getting comfortable with the standard exercises that will be used throughout the 12-week program. You'll start out using body weight and then progress to light weight. Each prep stage workout includes just two exercises, giving you plenty of time to focus on how you execute the move. Many of the moves in this stage are repeated throughout the plan, and that's intentional so you feel extra confident as you up the intensity in stages one through three.

Stage One: Mind-Muscle Connection

You could crank out a million dumbbell presses, but if you're not engaging the right muscles, you'll never see the results you want. That's why your first full phase in this strength-training journey will focus on actively thinking about what muscles you're using as you perform the moves in each workout. By the end of these four weeks, you'll feel totally locked in to each exercise, setting the stage for you to up the intensity—and your results.

Stage Two: Leveling Up

By stage two, you'll feel in control as you make your way through each exercise, which means you'll be ready to steadily increase the difficulty level. In stage two, progressive overload will be introduced—this is a fundamental principle in strength training where the difficulty level is gradually increased. We will do this by upping the intensity through more reps, the frequency of workouts, and number of exercises. This is how gains are made!

Stage Three: Bring the Heat!

Get ready to turn up the intensity in the final stage! We'll ramp up even further by incorporating advanced techniques and heavier weights to maximize muscle growth and definition.

Find Your Starting Point

Before you begin, I want you to note your base strength level. See how many reps of the following exercises you can do in one minute and how quickly you can complete a one-mile walk or run. Then, at the end of the program, return to this page, record your new results, and celebrate how far you've come.

EXERCISE	PRE-PLAN RESULTS	POST-PLAN RESULTS
Squat	In 1 min.:	In 1 min.:
Pushup	In 1 min.:	In 1 min.:
Situp	In 1 min.:	In 1 min.:
Burpee	In 1 min.:	In 1 min.:
Bonus: one-mile run or walk	Overall time:	Overall time:

With a focus on proper form, progressive overload training, balanced meals, and a touch of Nellbells Fitness's signature positivity alongside holistic health practices, this plan will guide you in transforming not only your body but also your mind.

Get ready to sweat, smile, and evolve!

Your 12-Week Dumbbell Strength-Training Plan

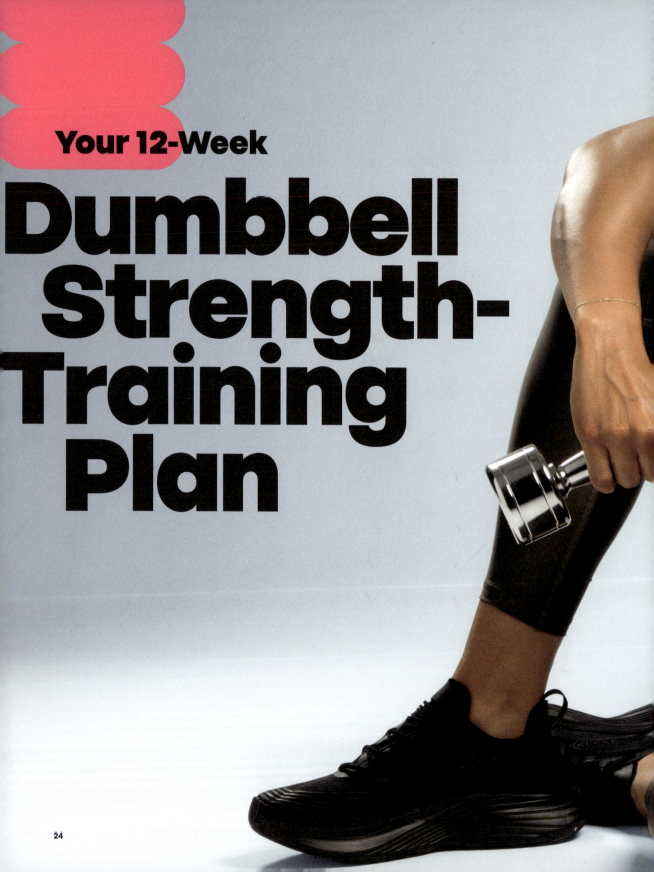

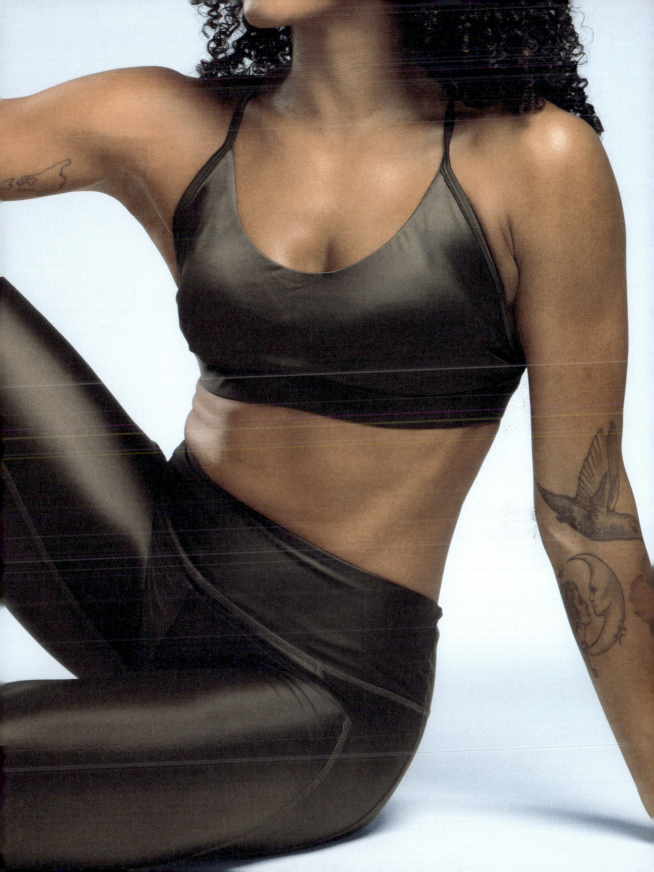

Your 12-Week Plan

PREP STAGE

Proper Form

NO MATTER WHAT your fitness level, the prep stage is a great place to start because over the next two weeks we will perform two exercises a day that will focus on the basics and use moves that will be included throughout the plan. This will get you ready to tackle the full plan with proper form.

For week one, all exercises are performed using only body weight. Week two is when light weight will be incorporated. Remember to experiment to find the right dumbbell weight for you using the guidance from page 16. Throughout the two weeks, I want you to move through each exercise with control and to pay close attention to form, as well as what you feel in your body as you go through the movement.

How to do the workout: Perform all sets of one exercise and then rest before starting the next exercise. Get moving again when you've caught your breath; your rest time between sets should not exceed 90 seconds in order to keep your heart rate up. For example, day one: perform 20 squats, rest, perform 20 squats, rest, perform 20 squats, rest, perform 12 pushups, rest, perform 12 pushups, rest, then perform the final set of 12 pushups…workout complete!

The tables in the next couple of pages outline the workouts and provides a space where you can track how you felt during each set and, when applicable, how much weight you used. If you need more room, use the notes section starting on page 207.

WEEK 1 • Body Weight Only

DAY	EXERCISE	WORK	SET 1	SET 2	SET 3
1	Squat (p. 190)	20 reps	2 min	1 min	1 min
	Pushup (p. 147)	12 reps	Modified	Modified	Regular!!
2	Glute Bridge (p. 183)	20 reps	✓	✓	✓
	Russian Twist (p. 178)	20 reps	✓	✓	✓
3	I-Y-T Raise (p. 145)	12 reps	✓	✓	✓
	Pushup (p. 147)	12 reps	✓	✓	✓
4	Rest				
5	Squat (p. 190)	20 reps	✓	✓	✓
	Deadbug (p. 176)	20 reps per side	✓	✓	✓
6	Pushup (p. 147)	12 reps	✓	✓	✓
	Glute Bridge (p. 183)	20 reps	✓	✓	✓
7	Rest				

Your 12-Week Plan

WEEK 2

DAY	EXERCISE	WORK	SET 1	SET 2	SET 3
8	Front Racked Squat (p. 194)	15 reps	✓	✓	✓
	Weighted Russian Twist (p. 179)	20 reps	✓	✓	✓
9	Dumbbell Single-Arm Row (p. 171)	12 reps per side	✓	✓	✓
	Deadbug (p. 176)	20 reps per side	✓	✓	✓
10	Rest				
11	Weighted Hip Thrust (p. 186)	20 reps	✓	✓	✓
	Overhead Triceps Extension (p. 152)	15 reps	✓	✓	✓
12	Chest Press (p. 159)	12 reps	✓	✓	✓
	Lateral Lunge (p. 188)	20 reps per side	✓	✓	
13	Rest				
14	Lateral Raise (p. 166)	12 reps			
	Shoulder Press (p. 163)	12 reps			

STAGE ONE

Mind-Muscle Connection

WELCOME TO THE FIRST 30 days of your 12-week strength-building program! Even though you're just getting started, you'll reap tons of benefits in these first few weeks that'll boost your fitness in the long run.

First, you'll cultivate one of the most powerful tools for building strength and optimizing your gains: the mind-muscle connection. This practice is just what it sounds like—using your mind to consciously engage the specific muscles being worked in a particular exercise. You can go through the motions, but are you actively engaging the muscles? For example, when you do a biceps curl, focus on squeezing the biceps on the concentric motion (this is when you raise the weight up) where you'll feel the muscles tighten and shorten. Then, focus on the eccentric motion (this is when you lower the weight down) where you'll feel the biceps elongate and stretch. Being intentional with your focus on mind-muscle connection will optimize your gains. If your muscles aren't properly engaged, it can increase your risk for injuries and muscle imbalances. Plus, you may end up using the wrong muscles, hindering your gains.

In stage one, you will build on the foundation of proper form and establish a strong mind-muscle connection to master controlled movements for strong technique.

You'll also establish the habit of getting your body moving (first with bodyweight exercises and then gradually with weights)—and isn't it so much easier to stick to your goals once they become second nature? It's said that it takes around 30 days to develop a habit, which is about how long you'll follow this first stage. You'll end this phase feeling stronger and excited to crush your weekly workouts for the rest of the plan—and beyond! Of course, you'll also get all those good-for-you strength-training benefits mentioned earlier, from improved balance to boosted mood.

You'll do three workouts per week this month, with one active recovery day (we'll have suggestions for you on these days throughout the plan, but feel free to switch things up according to what works best for you and your schedule) and three rest days. Pay extra attention to your body to practice your mind-muscle connection for all these movements. A lot of them work multiple parts of your body, but you can reference the exercise glossary on page 144 to see which muscle groups to focus on for each move.

Here's the suggested workout split:

| Workout 1 | Rest | Workout 2 | Rest | Workout 3 | Rest | Active Recovery |

You can switch up the workout split whatever way works best for you. If you find yourself constantly sore, try alternating your rest days between your workouts, similar to the above.

Your 12-Week Plan

WEEK 1 • At A Glance

- **DAY 1** — Leg Day
- **DAY 2** — Rest
- **DAY 3** — Upper Body Day
- **DAY 4** — Rest
- **DAY 5** — Shoulders and Chest Day
- **DAY 6** — Rest
- **DAY 7** — Active Recovery

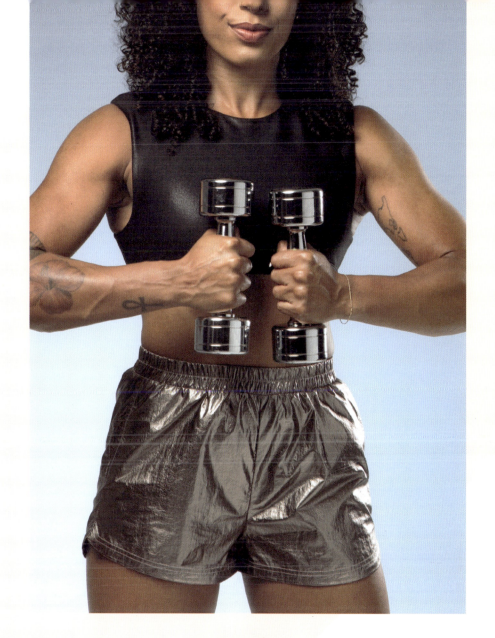

Your Plan This Week

In the following daily workouts, you'll see that we included **thumbnails so you can easily follow along** with the exercises this week. If you need more guidance, you can reference the **exercise glossary** (page number noted for each) to learn exactly how to do these moves. **And remember:** Track what weight you used for each move and each set in the space provided so you can make adjustments as you see fit and feel good about how you're progressing. **You got this!**

Your 12-Week Plan

Warm-up • Perform each exercise for 1 minute:

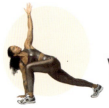
World's Greatest Stretch (p. 199)

Plank Walkout (p. 200)

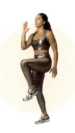
High Knee (p. 182)

WEEK 1 • DAY 1 • Leg Day

Rest 30 to 60 seconds between all sets

EXERCISE		WORK	SET 1
Weighted Hip Thrust (p. 186)		10 reps	
Dumbbell Swing (p. 198)		10 reps	
Russian Twist (p. 178)		10 reps	
Front Racked Squat (p. 194)		10 reps	

32 The Woman's Guide To Strength Training: Dumbbells

SET 2	SET 3
....	....
....	....
....	....

WEEK 1 • DAY 2 • Rest

You're probably experiencing some muscle soreness now. That dull ache you're feeling is called delayed-onset muscle soreness. It's different from an injury and it's actually a good sign that you've worked your muscles hard.

Stretching is a great way to work through stiffness and reduce discomfort. It'll also help you increase your range of motion, avoid muscle imbalances that can lead to injury, promote relaxation, and improve your posture, according to the American Council on Exercise (ACE).

Your 12-Week Plan

Warm-up • Perform each exercise for 1 minute:

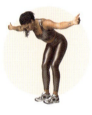
I-Y-T Raise (p. 145)

Thread the Needle (p. 146)

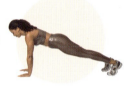
Pushup (p. 147)

WEEK 1 • DAY 3 • Upper Body Day

Rest 30 to 60 seconds between all sets

EXERCISE		WORK	SET 1
Reverse Fly (p. 154)		8 reps	
Dumbbell Single-Arm Row (p. 171)		8 reps per side	
Loaded Deadbug (p. 177)		8 reps per side	
Wide Biceps Curl (p. 150)		8 reps	

34 The Woman's Guide To Strength Training: Dumbbells

SET 2	SET 3
....	....
....	....
....	....

WEEK 1 • DAY 4 • Rest

If you do just one thing to help sore muscles, prioritize sleep. Deep sleep allows your body to release growth hormone, which is essential for building and repairing muscles, bones, and tissue, according to the Sleep Foundation.

Your 12-Week Plan

Warm-up • Perform each exercise for 1 minute:

Plank Walkout (p. 200)

Thread the Needle (p. 146)

Cat Cow (p. 144)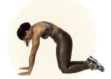

WEEK 1 • DAY 5 • Shoulders & Chest Day

Rest 30 to 60 seconds between all sets

EXERCISE		WORK	SET 1
Lateral Raise (p. 166)		10 reps	
Single-Arm Shoulder Press (p. 165)		10 reps per side	
Chest Press (p. 159)		10 reps	

36 The Woman's Guide To Strength Training: Dumbbells

SET 2	SET 3

WEEK 1 • DAY 6 • Rest

WEEK 1 • DAY 7 • Active Recovery

Adding a workout plan on top of your already busy schedule can feel overwhelming, so use Day 6 to unwind and focus on resting both your body and your mind. Ignore some chores (only for this day), walk the dog, or just dive into a book you've been meaning to read.

On Day 7, bounce back better by engaging in some active recovery, which is any low-intensity activity you can do while restoring and building muscle strength for future training. Take a leisurely bike ride or practice your breaststroke at the local community pool. Do what makes you feel good.

Your 12-Week Plan

WEEK 2 • At A Glance

- **DAY 8** — Leg Day
- **DAY 9** — Rest
- **DAY 10** — Back and Arms Day
- **DAY 11** — Rest
- **DAY 12** — Shoulders and Chest Day
- **DAY 13** — Rest
- **DAY 14** — Active Recovery

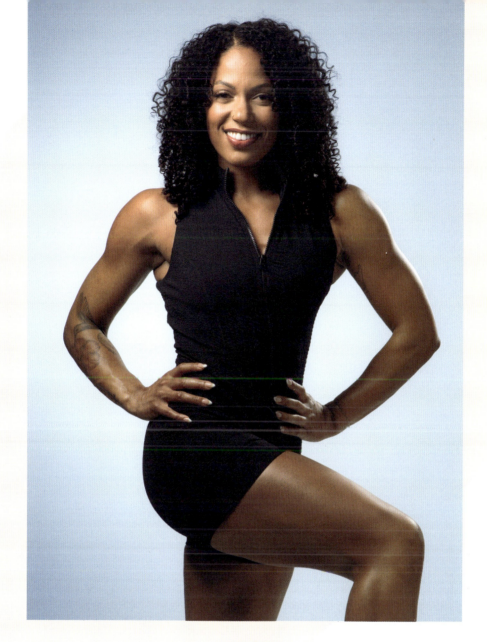

Your Plan This Week

In the following daily workouts, you'll see that we included **thumbnails so you can easily follow along** with the exercises this week. If you need more guidance, you can reference the **exercise glossary** (page number noted for each) to learn exactly how to do these moves. **And remember:** Track what weight you used for each move and each set in the space provided so you can make adjustments as you see fit and feel good about how you're progressing. **You got this!**

Your 12-Week Plan

Warm-up • Perform each exercise for 1 minute:

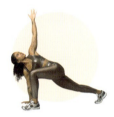
World's Greatest Stretch (p. 199)

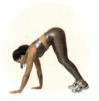
Plank Walkout (p. 200)

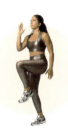
High Knee (p. 182)

WEEK 2 • DAY 8 • Leg Day

Rest 30 to 60 seconds between all sets

EXERCISE		WORK	SET 1
Lateral Lunge (p. 188)		10 reps per side	
Dumbbell Sumo Squat (p. 196)		10 reps	
Squat Jump (p. 197)		10 reps	

SET 2	SET 3
....	....
....	....
....	....

WEEK 2 • DAY 9 • Rest

Struggling to stay hydrated? Try eating your water. You can stave off dehydration by consuming more water-rich fruits and vegetables. Tomatoes, strawberries, watermelon, cantaloupe, and cucumbers are all great hydration helpers!

Your 12-Week Plan

Warm-up • Perform each exercise for 1 minute:

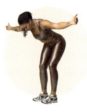
I-Y-T Raise (p. 145)

Thread the Needle (p. 146)

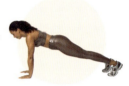
Pushup (p. 147)

WEEK 2 • DAY 10 • Back & Arms Day

Rest 30 to 60 seconds between all sets

EXERCISE		WORK	SET 1
Cross-Body Alternating Biceps Curl (p. 148)		8 reps	
Underhand Bent-Over Row (p. 172)		8 reps	
Overhead Triceps Extension (p. 152)		8 reps	

SET 2	SET 3
....	....
....	....

WEEK 2 • DAY 11 • Rest

Take a nice, long soak in the tub. While hard science is a bit soft on the muscle benefits of Epsom salts, we can attest: Placebo effect or not, an aromatic evening soak using Epsom salts plus a few drops of essential oils like eucalyptus and peppermint will leave you feeling oh-so-relaxed.

Your 12-Week Plan

Warm-up • Perform each exercise for 1 minute:

Plank Walkout (p. 200)

Thread the Needle (p. 146)

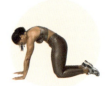
Cat Cow (p. 144)

WEEK 2 • DAY 12 • Shoulders & Chest Day

Rest 30 to 60 seconds between all sets

EXERCISE		WORK	SET 1
Lateral Raise (p. 166)		10 reps	
Kneeling Dumbbell Shoulder Press (p. 164)		10 reps	
Chest Fly (p. 153)		10 reps	
Zottman Curl (p. 151)		10 reps	

44 The Woman's Guide To Strength Training: Dumbbells

	SET 2	SET 3
	....	....
	....	....
	....	....

WEEK 2 • DAY 13 • Rest

WEEK 2 • DAY 14 • Active Recovery

As these workouts slowly ramp up in intensity, it's important to stay in tune with how your body feels. Meditating can be a bit intimidating at first, especially if you've never actually done it before, but on Day 13, try to focus on being more mindful of your body's needs and address them as needed.

On Day 14, follow it up with a yoga session. It's one of the best active recovery workouts you can do because it combines flexibility training with low-intensity, total-body strength training. Plus, it's relaxing and relieves stress. You really can't go wrong when you roll out that yoga mat!

Your 12-Week Plan

WEEK 3 • At A Glance

- **DAY 15** — Leg Day
- **DAY 16** — Rest
- **DAY 17** — Shoulders and Arms Day
- **DAY 18** — Rest
- **DAY 19** — Shoulders and Chest Day
- **DAY 20** — Rest
- **DAY 21** — Active Recovery

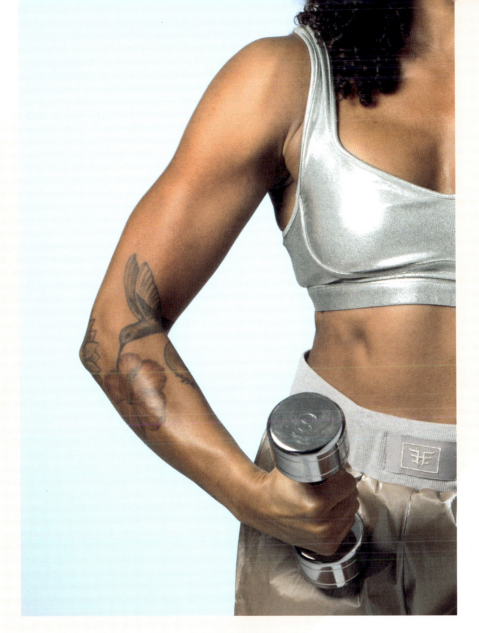

Your Plan This Week

In the following daily workouts, you'll see that we included **thumbnails so you can easily follow along** with the exercises this week. If you need more guidance, you can reference the **exercise glossary** (page number noted for each) to learn exactly how to do these moves. **And remember:** Track what weight you used for each move and each set in the space provided so you can make adjustments as you see fit and feel good about how you're progressing. **You got this!**

Your 12-Week Plan

Warm-up • Perform each exercise for 1 minute:

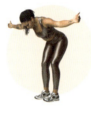

I-Y-T Raise (p. 145)

Thread the Needle (p. 146)

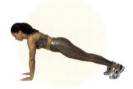

Pushup (p. 147)

WEEK 3 • DAY 15 • Leg Day

Rest 30 to 60 seconds between all sets

EXERCISE		WORK	SET 1
Squat Thruster (p. 206)		10 reps	
Goblet Squat (p. 193)		10 reps	
Lateral Lunge (p. 188)		10 reps per side	

48   The Woman's Guide To Strength Training: Dumbbells

SET 2 **SET 3**

WEEK 3 • DAY 16 • Rest

A good night's rest gives your muscles ample time to recover. If you're struggling to get quality sleep, think about adding a cup of herbal or decaffeinated tea to your nighttime ritual. Chamomile is a great choice due to its high levels of the antioxidant apigenin, which has been found to promote relaxation.

Your 12-Week Plan

Warm-up • Perform each exercise for 1 minute:

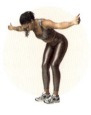
I-Y-T Raise (p. 145)

Thread the Needle (p. 146)

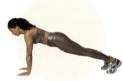
Pushup (p. 147)

WEEK 3 • DAY 17 • Shoulders & Arms Day

Rest 30 to 60 seconds between all sets

EXERCISE		WORK	SET 1
Hammer Curl (p. 149)		12 reps	
Upright Row (p. 173)		12 reps	
Skull Crusher (p. 174)		12 reps	
Toe Touch (p. 180)		20 reps	

SET 2 **SET 3**

WEEK 3 • DAY 18 • Rest

If you're like most Americans, you're probably taking in the bulk of your protein at dinner. But research shows that spreading protein consumption more evenly throughout the day helps better support your body's muscle repair and growth.

Try including a source of protein with every meal and snack you have throughout the day. It'll also keep you satiated so you don't end up snacking needlessly.

Your 12-Week Plan

Warm-up • Perform each exercise for 1 minute:

Plank Walkout (p. 200)   Thread the Needle (p. 146)   Cat Cow (p. 144)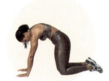

WEEK 3 • DAY 19 • Shoulders & Chest Day

Rest 30 to 60 seconds between all sets

EXERCISE		WORK	SET 1
Halo (p. 156)		10 reps	
Chest Fly (p. 153)		10 reps	
Bridge Chest Press (p. 158)		10 reps	
Russian Twist (p. 178)		20 reps	

52 The Woman's Guide To Strength Training: Dumbbells

SET 2	SET 3
....	....
....	....
....	....

WEEK 3 • DAY 20 • Rest

WEEK 3 • DAY 21 • Active Recovery

Scheduling in self-care is just as important as your workouts. On Day 20, do something that truly lights you up. Maybe that's taking an art class you've been meaning to check off your bucket list or trying a new restaurant that opened up. Find ways to re-energize ahead of this program's final week of Stage 1.

On Day 21, try Pilates. It's an excellent workout for active recovery days because it involves both stretching and low-intensity strength exercises that'll keep your blood circulating—without revving your heart rate—and leave you feeling long and limber.

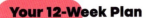

Your 12-Week Plan

WEEK 4 • At A Glance

- **DAY 22** — Leg Day
- **DAY 23** — Rest
- **DAY 24** — Back and Arms Day
- **DAY 25** — Rest
- **DAY 26** — Shoulders and Chest Day
- **DAY 27** — Rest
- **DAY 28** — Active Recovery

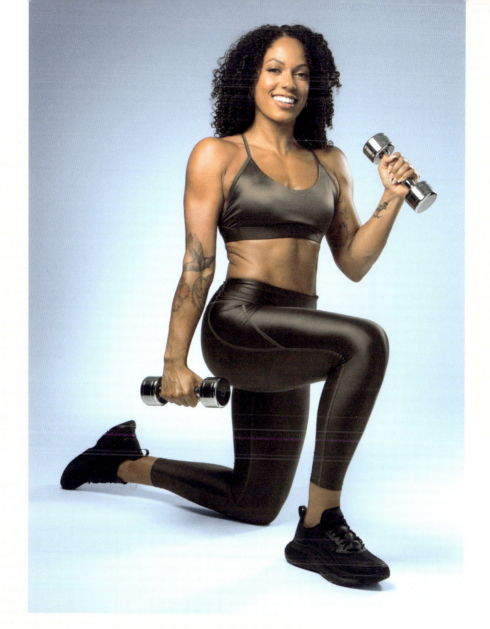

Your Plan This Week

In the following daily workouts, you'll see that we included **thumbnails so you can easily follow along** with the exercises this week. If you need more guidance, you can reference the **exercise glossary** (page number noted for each) to learn exactly how to do these moves. **And remember:** Track what weight you used for each move and each set in the space provided so you can make adjustments as you see fit and feel good about how you're progressing. **You got this!**

Your 12-Week Plan

Warm-up • Perform each exercise for 1 minute:

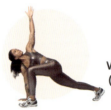
World's Greatest Stretch (p. 199)

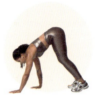
Plank Walkout (p. 200)

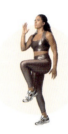
High Knee (p. 182)

WEEK 4 • DAY 22 • Leg Day

Rest 30 to 60 seconds between all sets

EXERCISE		WORK	SET 1
Two-Way Lunge (p. 189)		8 reps per side	
Romanian Deadlift (p. 184)		10 reps	
Dumbbell Swing (p. 198)		12 reps	

SET 2	SET 3
....	....
....	....

WEEK 4 • DAY 23 • Rest

Staying aotive and finding ways to keep your heart pumping is always a good thing, but if you're not feeling it today, that's perfectly fine too. You've been working hard, and that should come with some well-deserved rest. Take the day off and celebrate how far you've come. Just remember: Stay hydrated, eat well, and get enough sleep, and you'll hit the ground running tomorrow!

Your 12-Week Plan

Warm-up • Perform each exercise for 1 minute:

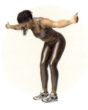
I-Y-T Raise (p. 145)

Thread the Needle (p. 146)

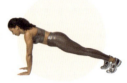
Pushup (p. 147)

WEEK 4 • DAY 24 • Back & Arms Day

Rest 30 to 60 seconds between all sets

EXERCISE		WORK	SET 1
Modified Burpee (p. 201)		8 reps	
Wood Chop (p. 181)		8 reps per side	
Gorilla Row (p. 170)		12 reps	
Alternating Reverse Fly (p. 155)		12 reps	

SET 2	SET 3
....	....
....	....
....	....

WEEK 4 • DAY 25 • Rest

Want a science-backed, all-natural remedy to reduce your recovery time after a tough workout? Try omega-3 fatty acids. Taking a daily fish-oil capsule may reduce soreness and ease inflammation 48 hours after a strength-training workout, a study in the *Clinical Journal of Sports Medicine* indicates. You can also incorporate more omega-3 rich foods into your diet: Salmon (which is also high in protein), rainbow trout, sardines, avocados, and walnuts are all great choices.

Your 12-Week Plan

Warm-up • Perform each exercise for 1 minute:

Plank Walkout (p. 200)

Thread the Needle (p. 146)

Cat Cow (p. 144)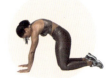

WEEK 4 • DAY 26 • Shoulders & Chest Day

Rest 30 to 60 seconds between all sets

EXERCISE		WORK	SET 1
Dumbbell Rainbow (p. 168)		10 reps	
Arnold Press (p. 157)		10 reps	
Alternating Chest Press (p. 160)		12 reps	
Loaded Deadbug (p. 177)		12 reps per side	

SET 2	SET 3
....	....
....	....
....	....

WEEK 4 • DAY 27 • Rest

WEEK 4 • DAY 28 • Active Recovery

Try making Day 27 an at-home spa day and add a few more steps to your normal shower routine. This may consist of exfoliating, shaving, applying hair mask or oil, and a scalp rub in addition to your shampoo, conditioner, and body wash. However you go about it, give your body a little extra TLC.

Foam rolling, which is basically self-massage, totally counts as active recovery. As you roll out your muscles on Day 28, you'll ward off soreness, boost your mobility, and help relieve stress (both mental and muscular) so you can recover faster between workouts.

Your 12-Week Plan

Congratulations, you've completed your first 28 days of the program!

The principles of proper form and mind-muscle connection that you've conquered are going to set you up for success as we level up to stage two and then bring the heat in stage three.

If you felt stage one was too challenging, I encourage you to repeat it before advancing, so that you're optimally prepared for what lies ahead. Mastering form and mind-muscle connection will get you the best results.

STAGE TWO
Leveling Up

It's time to kick things up a notch. One of the best ways to get results is to increase the difficulty of your training over time. This is known as progressive overload, and it can be done in a few different ways. You'll practice progressive overload in this stage using three methods. First, you'll bump up your total weekly workouts to four, eliminating one rest day. This increase in the frequency of workouts will have the biggest impact on your results because it's challenging the body's endurance. You're going to get stronger by increasing the frequency. In this stage, you'll also increase the number of repetitions during your sets to activate your muscles longer while keeping form tight. Because you are doing this from home with three dumbbell sets, it's best to start lighter and then work up to the heavier set. Last, you'll add variation with new exercises to target your muscles in new ways. For example, in stage one you performed front racked squats and in stage two you'll do staggered-stance front racked squats for the first time to challenge the same muscles in new ways. Variety keeps things interesting!

Here's the suggested workout split:

| Workout 1 | Workout 2 | Rest | Workout 3 | Active Recovery | Workout 4 | Rest |

WEEK 5 • At A Glance

- **DAY 29** — Leg Day
- **DAY 30** — Back and Arms Day
- **DAY 31** — Rest
- **DAY 32** — Shoulders and Chest Day
- **DAY 33** — Active Recovery
- **DAY 34** — Full Body Day
- **DAY 35** — Rest

Your 12-Week Plan

Warm-up • Perform each exercise for 1 minute:

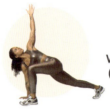
World's Greatest Stretch (p. 199)

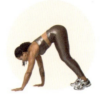
Plank Walkout (p. 200)

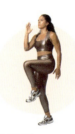
High Knee (p. 182)

WEEK 5 • DAY 29 • Leg Day

Rest 30 to 60 seconds between all sets

EXERCISE		WORK	SET 1
Weighted Hip Thrust (p. 186)		12 reps	
Dumbbell Swing (p. 198)		12 reps	
Side Plank Hip Dip (p. 175)		12 reps per side	
Front Racked Squat (p. 194)		12 reps	

SET 2	SET 3
....	....
....	....
....	....

Your Plan This Week

In these daily workouts, you'll see that we included **thumbnails so you can easily follow along** with the exercises this week. If you need more guidance, you can reference the **exercise glossary** (page number noted for each) to learn exactly how to do these moves. **And remember:** Track what weight you used for each move and each set in the space provided so you can make adjustments as you see fit and feel good about how you're progressing. **You got this!**

Your 12-Week Plan

Warm-up • Perform each exercise for 1 minute:

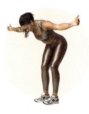
I-Y-T Raise (p. 145)

Thread the Needle (p. 146)

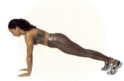
Pushup (p. 147)

WEEK 5 • DAY 30 • Back & Arms Day

Rest 30 to 60 seconds between all sets

EXERCISE		WORK	SET 1
Reverse Fly (p. 154)		10 reps	
Dumbbell Single-Arm Row (p. 171)		10 reps per side	
Loaded Deadbug (p. 177)		10 reps per side	
Wide Biceps Curl (p. 150)		10 reps	

SET 2	SET 3
....	....
....	....
....	....

WEEK 5 • DAY 31 • Rest

Close your eyes and take stock of how every part of your body feels. If you notice any imbalances, such as one side of your body feeling more relaxed than the other, focus more on stretching or massaging the side that feels tighter. This is a good opportunity to appreciate how far you've come in your journey.

Your 12-Week Plan

Warm-up • Perform each exercise for 1 minute:

Plank Walkout (p. 200)

Thread the Needle (p. 146)

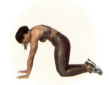
Cat Cow (p. 144)

WEEK 5 • DAY 32 • Shoulders & Chest Day

Rest 30 to 60 seconds between all sets

EXERCISE		WORK	SET 1
Alternating Front and Lateral Raise (p. 167)		10 reps	
Single-Arm Shoulder Press (p. 165)		10 reps per side	
Chest Press (p. 159)		10 reps	
Overhead Triceps Extension (p. 152)		10 reps	

SET 2	SET 3
....	....
....	....
....	....

WEEK 5 • DAY 33 • Active Recovery

Walking is a great active recovery option. Just getting outside for some fresh air will do wonders for not only your muscle recovery but also your mental health. And if you put a little pep in your step, it'll be a great cardio workout too!

Your 12-Week Plan

Warm-up • Perform each exercise for 1 minute:

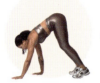
Plank Walkout (p. 200)

Thread the Needle (p. 146)

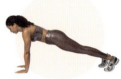
Pushup (p. 147)

WEEK 5 • DAY 34 • Full Body Day

Rest 30 to 60 seconds between all sets

EXERCISE		WORK	SET 1
Alternating Bent-Over Row (p. 169)		12 reps	
Squat Thruster (p. 206)		12 reps	
Dumbbell Speed Skater (p. 204)		12 reps	
Toe Touch (p. 180)		20 reps	

SET 2	SET 3
....	....
....	....
....	....

WEEK 5 • DAY 35 • Rest

Give your bones a boost. Strength training has been found to be the ultimate bone builder, but an unbalanced diet can leave you lacking in bone-fortifying vitamins and minerals. So load up on your bones' favorite mineral: calcium. Milk has always been a famous source of calcium, but it's not the only star. Add some of these calcium-rich foods into your diet: figs, artichokes, black beans, kale, almonds, and bok choy.

Your 12-Week Plan

WEEK 6 • At A Glance

- **DAY 36** — Leg Day
- **DAY 37** — Back and Arms Day
- **DAY 38** — Rest
- **DAY 39** — Shoulders and Chest Day
- **DAY 40** — Active Recovery
- **DAY 41** — Full Body Day
- **DAY 42** — Rest

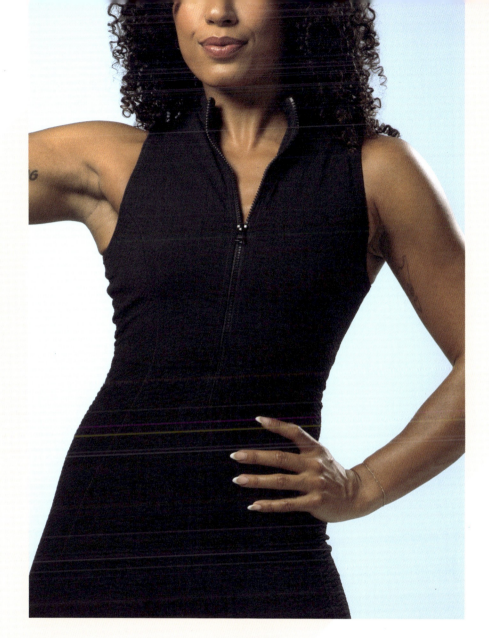

Your Plan This Week

In the following daily workouts, you'll see that we included **thumbnails so you can easily follow along** with the exercises this week. If you need more guidance, you can reference the **exercise glossary** (page number noted for each) to learn exactly how to do these moves. **And remember:** Track what weight you used for each move and each set in the space provided so you can make adjustments as you see fit and feel good about how you're progressing. **You got this!**

Your 12-Week Plan

Warm-up • Perform each exercise for 1 minute:

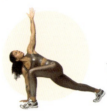
World's Greatest Stretch (p. 199)

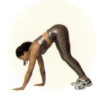
Plank Walkout (p. 200)

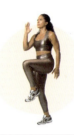
High Knee (p. 182)

WEEK 6 • DAY 36 • Leg Day

Rest 30 to 60 seconds between all sets

EXERCISE		WORK	SET 1
Staggered-Stance Front Racked Squat (p. 195)		8 reps per side	
Lateral Lunge (p. 188)		10 reps per side	
Dumbbell Sumo Squat (p. 196)		10 reps	
Squat Jump (p. 197)		10 reps	

74 The Woman's Guide To Strength Training: Dumbbells

SET 2	SET 3
....	....
....	....
....	....

Your 12-Week Plan

Warm-up • Perform each exercise for 1 minute:

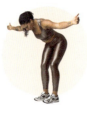
I-Y-T Raise (p. 145)

Thread the Needle (p. 146)

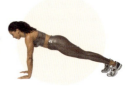
Pushup (p. 147)

WEEK 6 • DAY 37 • Back & Arms Day

Rest 30 to 60 seconds between all sets

EXERCISE		WORK	SET 1
Dumbbell Rainbow (p. 168)		10 reps	
Cross-Body Alternating Biceps Curl (p. 148)		10 reps	
Underhand Bent-Over Row (p. 172)		10 reps	
Overhead Triceps Extension (p. 152)		10 reps	

SET 2	SET 3
....	....
....	....
....	....

WEEK 6 • DAY 38 • Rest

Your muscles can't do anything without oxygen. You can easily **reduce stress** by harnessing something you do all day long—inhaling and exhaling.

Aim for six or seven slow, deep breaths per minute; inhale through your nose and exhale through your mouth while keeping your stomach relaxed. This helps calm your fight-or-flight engine and triggers your parasympathetic nervous system, which controls your rest and helps your muscles (and mind) unwind.

Your 12-Week Plan

Warm-up • Perform each exercise for 1 minute:

Plank Walkout (p. 200)

Thread the Needle (p. 146)

Cat Cow (p. 144)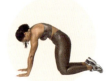

WEEK 6 • DAY 39 • Shoulders & Chest Day

Rest 30 to 60 seconds between all sets

EXERCISE		WORK	SET 1
Gator Press (p. 161)		10 reps	
Lateral Raise (p. 166)		10 reps	
Kneeling Dumbbell Shoulder Press (p. 164)		10 reps	
Chest Fly (p. 153)		10 reps	

SET 2	SET 3
....	....
....	....
....	....

WEEK 6 • DAY 40 • Active Recovery

Improve your range of motion and help nix aches and pains by doing mobility exercises. Think of them as little movements that can be incorporated into your daily routine—right when you wake up, while taking a quick break from sitting at your desk all day, or right before bed. These bite-size chunks of exercises will help minimize your risk of injury, improve joint health, reduce muscle soreness, and speed up the recovery process.

Your 12-Week Plan

Warm-up • Perform each exercise for 1 minute:

Plank Walkout (p. 200)

Thread the Needle (p. 146)

Pushup (p. 147)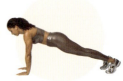

Rest 30 to 60 seconds between all sets

WEEK 6 • DAY 41 • Full Body Day

EXERCISE		WORK	SET 1
Reverse Lunge to Press (p. 202)		6 reps per side	
Modified Burpee (p. 201)		8 reps	
Skull Crusher (p. 174)		12 reps	
Russian Twist (p. 178)		20 reps	

SET 2	SET 3
....	....
....	....
....	....

WEEK 6 • DAY 42 • Rest

Want a super easy way to add protein to your diet? Most nuts contain 4 to 7 grams of plant-based protein per ounce. That's a decent boost for muscle repair and growth in just about ¼ cup—the perfect amount for stirring into yogurt, sprinkling on a grain bowl, or simply knocking back by the handful.

Go for peanuts, almonds, pistachios, and cashews (which are also great for immune support and muscle function, with their triple-threat bundle of zinc, copper, and magnesium).

Your 12-Week Plan

WEEK 7 • At A Glance

- **DAY 43** — Leg Day
- **DAY 44** — Back and Arms Day
- **DAY 45** — Rest
- **DAY 46** — Shoulders and Chest Day
- **DAY 47** — Active Recovery
- **DAY 48** — Full Body Day
- **DAY 49** — Rest

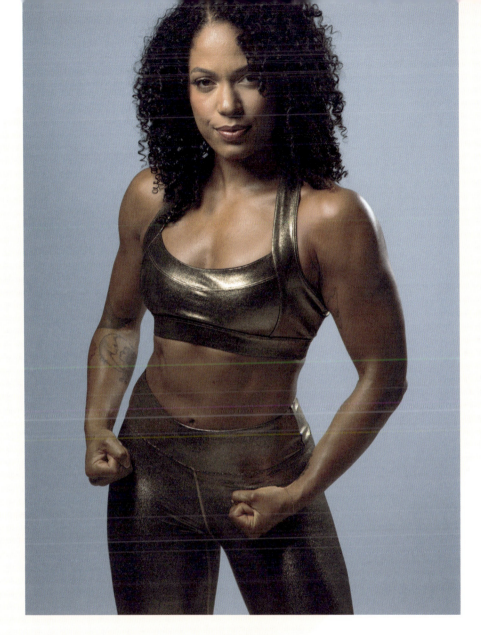

Your Plan This Week

In the following daily workouts, you'll see that we included **thumbnails so you can easily follow along** with the exercises this week. If you need more guidance, you can reference the **exercise glossary** (page number noted for each) to learn exactly how to do these moves. **And remember:** Track what weight you used for each move and each set in the space provided so you can make adjustments as you see fit and feel good about how you're progressing. **You got this!**

Your 12-Week Plan

Warm-up • Perform each exercise for 1 minute:

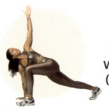
World's Greatest Stretch (p. 199)

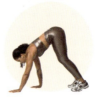
Plank Walkout (p. 200)

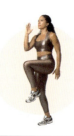
High Knee (p. 182)

WEEK 7 • DAY 43 • Leg Day

Rest 30 to 60 seconds between all sets

EXERCISE		WORK	SET 1
Back Squat (p. 191)		12 reps	
Squat Thruster (p. 206)		10 reps	
Russian Twist (p. 178)		20 reps	
Lateral Lunge (p. 188)		10 reps per side	

SET 2	SET 3
....	....
....	....
....	....

Your 12-Week Plan

Warm-up • Perform each exercise for 1 minute:

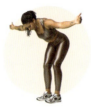
I-Y-T Raise (p. 145)

Thread the Needle (p. 146)

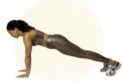
Pushup (p. 147)

WEEK 7 • DAY 44 • Back & Arms Day

Rest 30 to 60 seconds between all sets

EXERCISE		WORK	SET 1
Hammer Curl (p. 149)		12 reps	
Upright Row (p. 173)		12 reps	
Skull Crusher (p. 174)		12 reps	
Toe Touch (p. 180)		20 reps	

SET 2	SET 3
....	....
....	....
....	....

WEEK 7 • DAY 45 • Rest

The first moments of a new day can have a big impact on your next 24 hours. Instead of rushing into a busy routine and hustling to be productive right away, why not take this opportunity to calm your nervous system by prioritizing self-care and cultivating mindfulness?

It doesn't have to be a whole production. It can be as simple as journaling, sitting outside and watching the sun rise, savoring the smell of coffee brewing, or listening to music while taking a relaxing shower.

Your 12-Week Plan

Warm-up • Perform each exercise for 1 minute:

Plank Walkout (p. 200)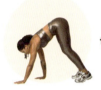
Thread the Needle (p. 146)
Cat Cow (p. 144)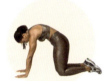

WEEK 7 • DAY 46 • Shoulders & Chest Day

Rest 30 to 60 seconds between all sets

EXERCISE	WORK	SET 1
Halo (p. 156)	12 reps	
Chest Fly (p. 153)	12 reps	
Dumbbell Seesaw Press (p. 162)	12 reps	
Loaded Deadbug (p. 177)	10 reps per side	

SET 2	SET 3
....	....
....	....
....	....

WEEK 7 • DAY 47 • Active Recovery

Riding a bike, stationary or otherwise, definitely qualifies as an active recovery workout. This low-impact, low-intensity exercise allows you to work on your muscle endurance and get in some steady-state cardio. Just be sure to maintain a leisurely-to-moderate pace.

Your 12-Week Plan

Warm-up • Perform each exercise for 1 minute:

Plank Walkout (p. 200)

Thread the Needle (p. 146)

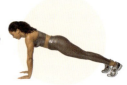
Pushup (p. 147)

WEEK 7 • DAY 48 • Full Body Day

Rest 30 to 60 seconds between all sets

EXERCISE		WORK	SET 1
Wide Biceps Curl (p. 150)		12 reps	
Goblet Squat (p. 193)		10 reps	
Side Plank Hip Dip (p. 175)		12 reps per side	
Back Squat (p. 191)		12 reps	

SET 2	SET 3
....	....
....	....
....	....

WEEK 7 • DAY 49 • Rest

Ever been told to apply ice or heat to an injury? That repetitive application of cold and then heat in an alternating fashion is called contrast therapy: The cold helps reduce swelling while the heat promotes blood flow and removes waste products such as carbon dioxide and lactic acid.

Try using a product like Icy Hot. The rub-on ointment utilizes the principles of contrast therapy, providing both cooling and heating sensations to relieve muscle soreness.

Your 12-Week Plan

WEEK 8 • At A Glance

- **DAY 50** — Leg Day
- **DAY 51** — Back and Arms Day
- **DAY 52** — Rest
- **DAY 53** — Shoulders and Chest Day
- **DAY 54** — Active Recovery
- **DAY 55** — Full Body Day
- **DAY 56** — Rest

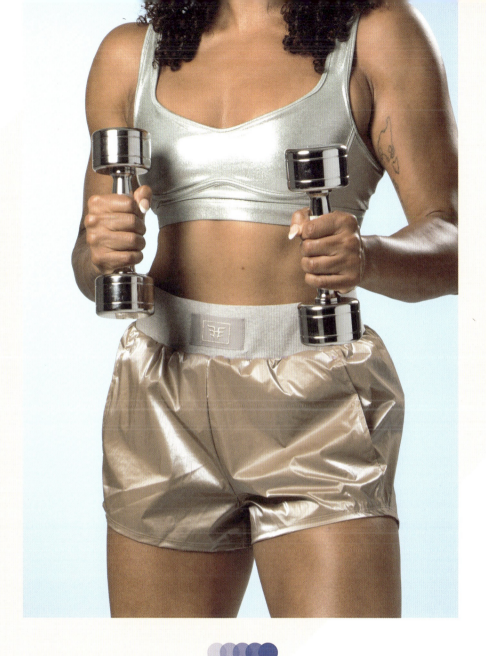

Your Plan This Week

In the following daily workouts, you'll see that we included **thumbnails so you can easily follow along** with the exercises this week. If you need more guidance, you can reference the **exercise glossary** (page number noted for each) to learn exactly how to do these moves. **And remember:** Track what weight you used for each move and each set in the space provided so you can make adjustments as you see fit and feel good about how you're progressing. **You got this!**

Your 12-Week Plan

Warm-up • Perform each exercise for 1 minute:

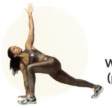
World's Greatest Stretch (p. 199)

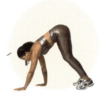
Plank Walkout (p. 200)

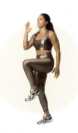
High Knee (p. 182)

WEEK 8 • DAY 50 • Leg Day

Rest 30 to 60 seconds between all sets

EXERCISE	WORK	SET 1
Two-Way Lunge (p. 189)	8 reps per side	
Staggered-Stance Deadlift (p. 185)	10 reps per side	
Dumbbell Swing (p. 198)	12 reps	
Loaded Deadbug (p. 177)	10 reps per side	

The Woman's Guide To Strength Training: Dumbbells

SET 2	SET 3
....	....
....	....
....	....

Your 12-Week Plan

Warm-up • Perform each exercise for 1 minute:

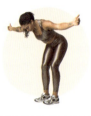
I-Y-T Raise (p. 145)

Thread the Needle (p. 146)

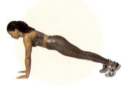
Pushup (p. 147)

Rest 30 to 60 seconds between all sets

WEEK 8 • DAY 51 • Back & Arms Day

EXERCISE		WORK	SET 1
Modified Burpee (p. 201)		10 reps	
Wood Chop (p. 181)		10 reps per side	
Gorilla Row (p. 170)		12 reps	
Alternating Reverse Fly (p. 155)		12 reps	

SET 2	SET 3
....	....
....	....
....	....

WEEK 8 • DAY 52 • Rest

When it comes to snacking, the baseline for a high-protein snack is about 6 or 7 grams of protein. After a tough workout though, it's good to increase the protein content of your snack to help with muscle repair. Aim for 10 to 15 grams.

What does that look like? A serving of string cheese with a handful of nuts, cottage cheese with a bit of your favorite fruit preserves, or a slice of whole-grain toast with your favorite nut butter.

Your 12-Week Plan

Warm-up • Perform each exercise for 1 minute:

Plank Walkout (p. 200)
Thread the Needle (p. 146)
Cat Cow (p. 144)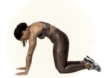

WEEK 8 • DAY 53 • Shoulders & Chest Day

Rest 30 to 60 seconds between all sets

EXERCISE		WORK	SET 1
Dumbbell Rainbow (p. 168)		10 reps	
Arnold Press (p. 157)		10 reps	
Alternating Chest Press (p. 160)		12 reps	
Toe Touch (p. 180)		20 reps	

SET 2	SET 3
....	....
....	....
....	....

WEEK 8 • DAY 54 • Active Recovery

Consider taking a dip in a pool today as your active recovery. Swimming isn't just good for your circulation; it's also a light form of resistance training that's easy on your joints. Try going at an easy pace to reap the active recovery benefits.

Your 12-Week Plan

Warm-up • Perform each exercise for 1 minute:

 Plank Walkout (p. 200)

 Thread the Needle (p. 146)

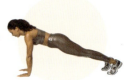 Pushup (p. 147)

WEEK 8 • DAY 55 • Full Body Day

Rest 30 to 60 seconds between all sets

EXERCISE		WORK	SET 1
Cross-Body Alternating Biceps Curl (p. 148)		10 reps	
Gator Press (p. 161)		10 reps	
Weighted Hip Thrust (p. 186)		15 reps	
Squat and Snatch (p. 205)		12 reps per side	

100 The Woman's Guide To Strength Training: Dumbbells

SET 2	SET 3
....	....
....	....
....	....

WEEK 8 • DAY 56 • Rest

Take this time to do a mental reset. Working out requires serious focus and mental fortitude, so give your mind a break. Remember that rest days should include whatever brings you joy—reading a captivating book, whipping up a favorite dessert, or spending time with loved ones—so you can go into the next phase of this program feeling refreshed and energized.

Your 12-Week Plan

Even with more workouts, you got it done! Way to work.

I'm sure there were days when you felt super sore, or maybe life got in the way, but you figured out how to prioritize your workouts and squeeze in an extra one each week. Give yourself a pat on the back for rising to the occasion during stage two of leveling up!

Now that it's time for the final check-in, do you feel like you're ready to push yourself a little harder? If so, continue on to stage three. If not, that's totally okay! It's called a fitness journey for a reason, because it takes time to get into the rhythm and build strength. I encourage you to revisit stage two and make it a priority to plan out your workouts for the week. Enjoy the process!

STAGE THREE

Bring the Heat!

Get ready to take it up a notch in the final stage! In these final four weeks, you'll ramp up the intensity even further by incorporating advanced techniques and heavier weights to maximize muscle growth and definition. These will be your most challenging workouts, but all your hard work the last 56 days has prepared you for it.

Some of the new techniques are:

SUPERSETS: This is a strength-training technique where you perform two exercises back-to-back with little to no rest between sets. For example, you would perform 10 reps of exercise one then immediately go into exercise two to perform 10 reps and then rest. Supersets are great for maximizing your gains because you can do more in less time, and they add cardio with the minimal rests between sets, which makes your heart rate go up.

PYRAMID SETS: To do these, you increase the dumbbell weight for each set and decrease the number of reps as you go up in weight. For example, if you are performing three sets of chest presses, you would start with 12 reps at a lighter weight, then your next set would be 10 reps at a heavier weight, and your last set would be 8 reps at the heaviest weight you can do. As the dumbbell weight goes up, the number of reps goes down. Pyramid sets are great for fatiguing the muscle fibers while pushing your limits safely and maintaining proper form—sometimes you're able to lift heavier than you thought possible because the reps in a set start to go down.

Are you ready to level up? Remember, it's mind over matter—you got this!

WEEK 9 • At A Glance

- **DAY 57** — Leg Day
- **DAY 58** — Back and Arms Day
- **DAY 59** — Rest
- **DAY 60** — Shoulders and Arms Day
- **DAY 61** — Active Recovery
- **DAY 62** — Full Body Day
- **DAY 63** — Rest

Your 12-Week Plan

Warm-up • Perform each exercise for 1 minute:

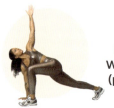
World's Greatest Stretch (p. 199)

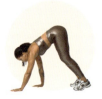
Plank Walkout (p. 200)

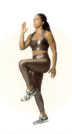
High Knee (p. 182)

WEEK 9 • DAY 57 • Leg Day

Rest 30 to 60 seconds between all sets

EXERCISE		WORK	SET 1
Weighted Hip Thrust (p. 186)		20 reps, then 15, then 10	
Dumbbell Swing (p. 198)		15 reps	
Side Plank Hip Dip (p. 175)		15 reps per side	
Front Racked Squat (p. 194)		15 reps	

104   The Woman's Guide To Strength Training: Dumbbells

SET 2	SET 3
....	....
....	....
....	....

Your Plan This Week

In these daily workouts, you'll see that we included **thumbnails so you can easily follow along** with the exercises this week. If you need more guidance, you can reference the **exercise glossary** (page number noted for each) to learn exactly how to do these moves. **And remember:** Track what weight you used for each move and each set in the space provided so you can make adjustments as you see fit and feel good about how you're progressing. **You got this!**

Your 12-Week Plan

Warm-up • Perform each exercise for 1 minute:

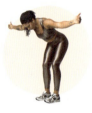

I-Y-T Raise (p. 145)

Thread the Needle (p. 146)

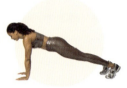

Pushup (p. 147)

WEEK 9 • DAY 58 • Back & Arms Day

Rest 30 to 60 seconds between all sets

EXERCISE		WORK	SET 1
Reverse Fly (p. 154)		12 reps	
Dumbbell Single-Arm Row (p. 171)		12 reps per side, then 10, then 8	
Loaded Deadbug (p. 177)		12 reps per side	
Wide Biceps Curl (p. 150)		12 reps	

106 The Woman's Guide To Strength Training: Dumbbells

SET 2	SET 3
....	....
....	....
....	....

WEEK 9 • DAY 59 • Rest

Carve out some time to lie down for a quick 30 minutes of shut-eye today. A short daytime power nap has been shown to help rejuvenate the body quickly, as deep, slow-wave sleep can restore energy—including energy needed for recovery processes to take place.

Your 12-Week Plan

Warm-up • Perform each exercise for 1 minute:

Plank Walkout (p. 200)

Thread the Needle (p. 146)

Cat Cow (p. 144)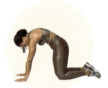

WEEK 9 • DAY 60 • Shoulders & Arms Day

Rest 30 to 60 seconds between all sets

EXERCISE		WORK	SET 1
Alternating Front and Lateral Raise (p. 167)		10 reps	
Single-Arm Shoulder Press (p. 165)		12 reps per side, then 10, then 8	
Russian Twist (p. 178)		20 reps	
Overhead Triceps Extension (p. 152)		12 reps	

SET 2	SET 3
....	....
....	....
....	....

WEEK 9 • DAY 61 • Active Recovery

Try a rowing machine workout. Rowing engages up to 86 percent of your muscles at once. Basically, it works your whole body and can really rev your heart rate. It also puts way less stress on your joints than running does. Keep to a steady pace with an effort level of 4 or 5 out of 10 and this low-impact workout can be a solid recovery activity.

Your 12-Week Plan

Warm-up • Perform each exercise for 1 minute:

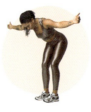
I-Y-T Raise (p. 145)

Thread the Needle (p. 146)

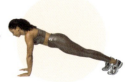
Pushup (p. 147)

WEEK 9 • DAY 62 • Full Body Day

Rest 30 to 60 seconds between all sets

EXERCISE		WORK	SET 1
SUPERSET 1: Zottman Curl (p. 151)		12 reps	
Chest Press (p. 159)		12 reps	
SUPERSET 2: Squat and Snatch (p. 205)		12 reps per side	
Dumbbell Speed Skater (p. 204)		20 reps	

SET 2   **SET 3**

WEEK 9 • DAY 63 • Rest

You already know that consuming enough protein is super important for building and maintaining muscle. But if you're having a hard time getting your fill of the macro from real foods, supplement with protein powder.

Get creative with all the ways you can incorporate protein powder into your meals: Blend it in your favorite smoothie, throw it into your go-to pancake mix, or puree it with some frozen bananas to make a protein ice cream.

Your 12-Week Plan

WEEK 10 • At A Glance

- **DAY 64** — Leg Day
- **DAY 65** — Back and Arms Day
- **DAY 66** — Rest
- **DAY 67** — Shoulders and Chest Day
- **DAY 68** — Active Recovery
- **DAY 69** — Full Body Day
- **DAY 70** — Rest

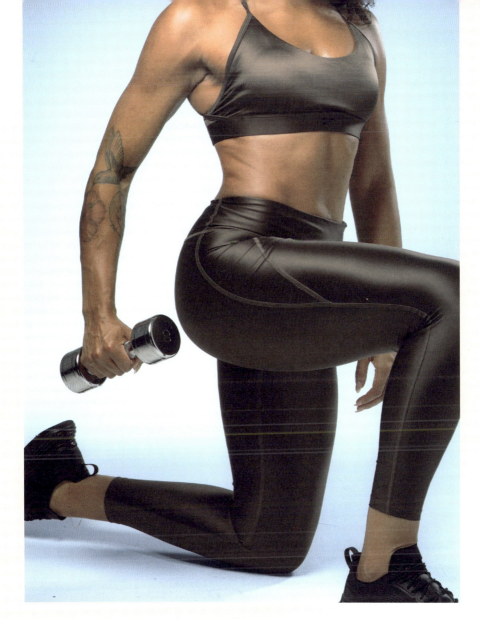

Your Plan This Week

In the following daily workouts, you'll see that we included **thumbnails so you can easily follow along** with the exercises this week. If you need more guidance, you can reference the **exercise glossary** (page number noted for each) to learn exactly how to do these moves. **And remember:** Track what weight you used for each move and each set in the space provided so you can make adjustments as you see fit and feel good about how you're progressing. **You got this!**

Your 12-Week Plan

Warm-up • Perform each exercise for 1 minute:

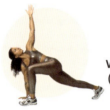
World's Greatest Stretch (p. 199)

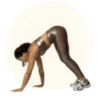
Plank Walkout (p. 200)

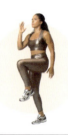
High Knee (p. 182)

WEEK 10 • DAY 64 • Leg Day

Rest 30 to 60 seconds between all sets

EXERCISE		WORK	SET 1
Staggered-Stance Front Racked Squat (p. 195)		8 reps per side	
Lateral Lunge (p. 188)		10 reps per side	
Dumbbell Sumo Squat (p. 196)		10 reps	
Deficit Reverse Lunge (p. 187)		8 reps per side	

SET 2	SET 3
....	....
....	....
....	....

Your 12-Week Plan

Warm-up • Perform each exercise for 1 minute:

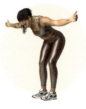
I-Y-T Raise (p. 145)

Thread the Needle (p. 146)

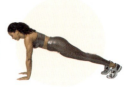
Pushup (p. 147)

WEEK 10 • DAY 65 • Back & Arms Day

Rest 30 to 60 seconds between all sets

EXERCISE		WORK	SET 1
Dumbbell Rainbow (p. 168)		10 reps	
Cross-Body Alternating Biceps Curl (p. 148)		10 reps	
Underhand Bent-Over Row (p. 172)		12 reps, then 10, then 8	
Overhead Triceps Extension (p. 152)		10 reps	

SET 2	SET 3
....	....
....	....
....	....

WEEK 10 • DAY 66 • Rest

Remember that day you absolutely crushed your shoulder and arm workout and felt like a superhero afterward? Put that memory top of mind the next time you're staring down the dumbbells.

In one University of New Hampshire study, participants asked to think about positive exercise memories had higher levels of subsequent exercise than those who didn't take that trip down memory lane. In other words, the more you associate positive emotions with working out, the more likely you are to show up.

Your 12-Week Plan

Warm-up • Perform each exercise for 1 minute:

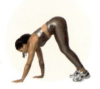
Plank Walkout (p. 200)

Thread the Needle (p. 146)

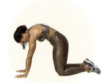
Cat Cow (p. 144)

WEEK 10 • DAY 67 • Shoulders & Chest Day

Rest 30 to 60 seconds between all sets

EXERCISE		WORK	SET 1
Gator Press (p. 161)		10 reps	
Lateral Raise (p. 166)		10 reps	
Kneeling Dumbbell Shoulder Press (p. 164)		12 reps, then 10, then 8	
Chest Fly (p. 153)		10 reps	

SET 2	SET 3
....	....
....	....
....	....

WEEK 10 • DAY 68 • Active Recovery

Hitting the trail is an opportunity to decompress, soak up fresh air, and give your muscles a chance to recover while still keeping them engaged. Plus, time spent off the beaten track can do everything from lessening depression to boosting heart and immune health, per research in the *American Journal of Lifestyle Medicine*. So lace up your hiking boots and think of your outing as a moving meditation.

Your 12-Week Plan

Warm-up • Perform each exercise for 1 minute:

Plank Walkout (p. 200)

Thread the Needle (p. 146)

Pushup (p. 147)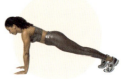

WEEK 10 • DAY 69 • Full Body Day

Rest 30 to 60 seconds between all sets

EXERCISE		WORK	SET 1
SUPERSET 1: Halo (p. 156)		12 reps	
Squat Jump (p. 197)		12 reps	
SUPERSET 2: Loaded Deadbug (p. 177)		12 reps per side	
Modified Devil Press (p. 203)		10 reps	

120 The Woman's Guide To Strength Training: Dumbbells

SET 2	SET 3

WEEK 10 • DAY 70 • Rest

Is delayed-onset muscle soreness leaving you restless come bedtime? Magnesium is a mineral that can help your muscles relax. It also breaks down protein more efficiently for muscle repair and function and converts it into chemicals that help you feel sleepy.

Before you go for an over-the-counter magnesium supplement, though, turn to whole foods to get those quality Zs. Some of the best sources include pumpkin seeds, chia seeds, almonds, spinach, and black beans.

Your 12-Week Plan

WEEK 11 • At A Glance

- **DAY 71** — Leg Day
- **DAY 72** — Back and Arms Day
- **DAY 73** — Rest
- **DAY 74** — Shoulders and Chest Day
- **DAY 75** — Active Recovery
- **DAY 76** — Full Body Day
- **DAY 77** — Rest

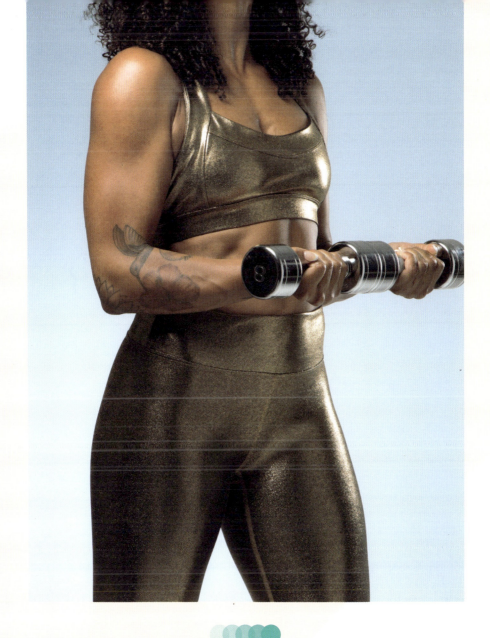

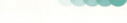

Your Plan This Week

In the following daily workouts, you'll see that we included **thumbnails so you can easily follow along** with the exercises this week. If you need more guidance, you can reference the **exercise glossary** (page number noted for each) to learn exactly how to do these moves. **And remember:** Track what weight you used for each move and each set in the space provided so you can make adjustments as you see fit and feel good about how you're progressing. **You got this!**

Your 12-Week Plan

Warm-up • Perform each exercise for 1 minute:

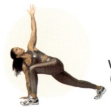
World's Greatest Stretch (p. 199)

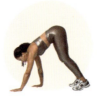
Plank Walkout (p. 200)

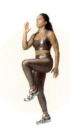
High Knee (p. 182)

WEEK 11 • DAY 71 • Leg Day

Rest 30 to 60 seconds between all sets

EXERCISE		WORK	SET 1
Bulgarian Split Squat (p. 192)		8 reps per side	
Back Squat (p. 191)		12 reps, then 10, then 8	
Squat Thruster (p. 206)		10 reps	
Russian Twist (p. 178)		20 reps	

SET 2	SET 3
....	....
....	....
....	....

Your 12-Week Plan

Warm-up • Perform each exercise for 1 minute:

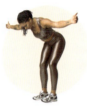

I-Y-T Raise (p. 145)

Thread the Needle (p. 146)

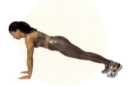

Pushup (p. 147)

WEEK 11 • DAY 72 • Back & Arms Day

Rest 30 to 60 seconds between all sets

EXERCISE		WORK	SET 1
Hammer Curl (p. 149)		12 reps	
Upright Row (p. 173)		12 reps, then 10, then 8	
Skull Crusher (p. 174)		12 reps	
Toe Touch (p. 180)		20 reps	

126 The Woman's Guide To Strength Training: Dumbbells

SET 2	SET 3
....	....
....	....
....	....

WEEK 11 • DAY 73 • Rest

By now you're probably feeling a lot stronger than you did when you started the program—and maybe even ready to hit the weights every day! But remember: Your body needs time to recover.

You can be strategic about your rest days. Since yesterday and tomorrow are both upper-body workouts, recovery today can include an easy, low-impact lower-body workout that works an entirely different set of muscles.

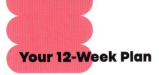

Your 12-Week Plan

Warm-up • Perform each exercise for 1 minute:

Plank Walkout (p. 200)   Thread the Needle (p. 146)   Cat Cow (p. 144)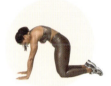

WEEK 11 • DAY 74 • Shoulders & Chest Day

Rest 30 to 60 seconds between all sets

EXERCISE		WORK	SET 1
Halo (p. 156)		12 reps	
Chest Fly (p. 153)		12 reps	
Dumbbell Seesaw Press (p. 162)		12 reps, then 10, then 8	
Loaded Deadbug (p. 177)		12 reps per side	

SET 2	SET 3
....	....
....	....
....	....

WEEK 11 • DAY 75 • Active Recovery

If you don't know how to swim or just aren't a fan of the backstroke, give water aerobics a try. Thanks to the resistance of the water, you can reap cardio and strength benefits without even hitting the deep end. Try pool exercises such as dips, scissor kicks, and jogging in place to mix things up.

Your 12-Week Plan

Warm-up • Perform each exercise for 1 minute:

Plank Walkout (p. 200)

Thread the Needle (p. 146)

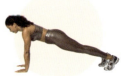
Pushup (p. 147)

WEEK 11 • DAY 76 • Full Body Day

Rest 90 seconds between supersets

EXERCISE		WORK	SET 1
SUPERSET 1: Dumbbell Speed Skater (p. 204)		20 reps	
Squat and Snatch (p. 205)		12 reps per side	
SUPERSET 2: Lateral Lunge (p. 188)		10 reps per side	
Bridge Chest Press (p. 158)		12 reps, then 10, then 8	

130 The Woman's Guide To Strength Training: Dumbbells

SET 2	SET 3

WEEK 11 • DAY 77 • Rest

Carbs have gotten a bad rap since the rise of keto, but they play a critical role in fueling your workouts. Apart from being your body's essential source of energy, "good" carbs have high fiber content (to keep you full longer), muscle-building protein, and a whole host of vitamins and antioxidants.

Try to avoid carbs that are highly processed and contain added sugars, and aim to incorporate whole-food carbs, such as quinoa, oatmeal, chickpeas, bananas, sweet potatoes, and carrots, into a balanced diet.

Your 12-Week Plan

WEEK 12 • At A Glance

- **DAY 78** — Leg Day
- **DAY 79** — Back and Arms Day
- **DAY 80** — Rest
- **DAY 81** — Shoulders and Chest Day
- **DAY 82** — Active Recovery
- **DAY 83** — Full Body Day
- **DAY 84** — Rest

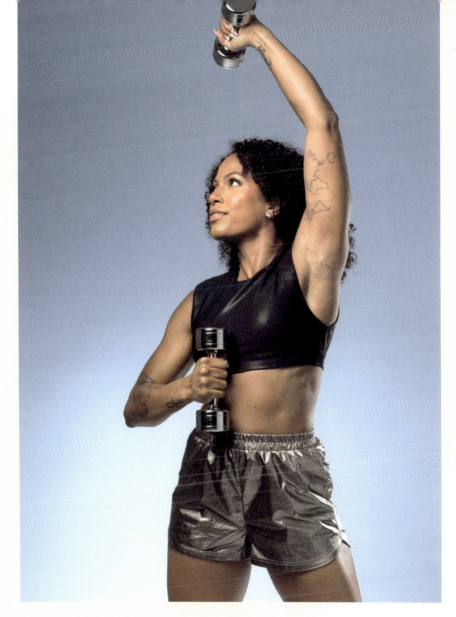

Your Plan This Week

In the following daily workouts, you'll see that we included **thumbnails so you can easily follow along** with the exercises this week. If you need more guidance, you can reference the **exercise glossary** (page number noted for each) to learn exactly how to do these moves. **And remember:** Track what weight you used for each move and each set in the space provided so you can make adjustments as you see fit and feel good about how you're progressing. **You got this!**

Your 12-Week Plan

Warm-up • Perform each exercise for 1 minute:

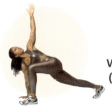 World's Greatest Stretch (p. 199)

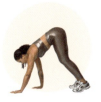 Plank Walkout (p. 200)

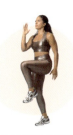 High Knee (p. 182)

WEEK 12 • DAY 78 • Leg Day

Rest 30 to 60 seconds between all sets

EXERCISE		WORK	SET 1
Two-Way Lunge (p. 189)		8 reps per side	
Staggered-Stance Deadlift (p. 185)		12 reps per side, then 10, then 8	
Dumbbell Swing (p. 198)		12 reps	
Loaded Deadbug (p. 177)		12 reps per side	

134 The Woman's Guide To Strength Training: Dumbbells

SET 2	SET 3
....	....
....	....
....	....

Your 12-Week Plan

Warm-up • Perform each exercise for 1 minute:

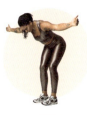
I-Y-T Raise (p. 145)

Thread the Needle (p. 146)

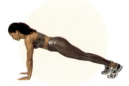
Pushup (p. 147)

WEEK 12 • DAY 79 • Back & Arms Day

Rest 30 to 60 seconds between all sets

EXERCISE		WORK	SET 1
Gorilla Row (p. 170)		12 reps, then 10, then 8	
Modified Burpee (p. 201)		10 reps	
Wood Chop (p. 181)		12 reps per side	
Alternating Reverse Fly (p. 155)		12 reps	

136 The Woman's Guide To Strength Training: Dumbbells

SET 2	SET 3
....	....
....	....
....	....

WEEK 12 • DAY 80 • Rest

Give yourself the right kind of pep talk. Research suggests that talking to yourself in the second person ("you") can actually be more effective than chatting yourself up in the first person ("I"). So the next time you're feeling sluggish, tell yourself, "You've got this!" instead of "I can do this."

Your 12-Week Plan

Warm-up • Perform each exercise for 1 minute:

Plank Walkout (p. 200)

Thread the Needle (p. 146)

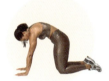
Cat Cow (p. 144)

WEEK 12 • DAY 81 • Shoulders & Chest Day

Rest 30 to 60 seconds between all sets

EXERCISE		WORK	SET 1
Dumbbell Rainbow (p. 168)		10 reps	
Alternating Chest Press (p. 160)		12 reps, then 10, then 8	
Arnold Press (p. 157)		10 reps	
Toe Touch (p. 180)		20 reps	

138 The Woman's Guide To Strength Training: Dumbbells

SET 2	SET 3
....	....
....	....
....	....

WEEK 12 • DAY 82 • Active Recovery

Look for ways to incorporate extra movement into your day to clear your mind or just to add more steps to your daily count. A few ideas to get you started:

• Take the stairs instead of getting on the elevator at work.

• Walk the longer route to your favorite coffee shop.

• Shop for groceries in person instead of ordering them online.

Your 12-Week Plan

Warm-up • Perform each exercise for 1 minute:

Plank Walkout (p. 200)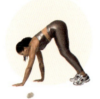

Thread the Needle (p. 146)

Pushup (p. 147)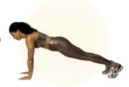

WEEK 12 • DAY 83 • Full Body Day

Rest 90 seconds between supersets

EXERCISE		WORK	SET 1
SUPERSET 1:			
Modified Devil Press (p. 203)		10 reps	
Side Plank Hip Dip (p. 175)		12 reps per side	
SUPERSET 2:			
Cross-Body Alternating Biceps Curl (p. 148)		10 reps	
Bulgarian Split Squat (p. 192)		8 reps per side	

140 The Woman's Guide To Strength Training: Dumbbells

SET 2	SET 3
....	....

WEEK 12 • DAY 84 • Rest

Congratulations! You crushed it! Now treat yourself to a well-deserved massage.

You already know that a solid rubdown has impressive health perks, like better blood circulation, amped immunity, and anxiety relief. But the true magic of a massage is that it can trigger powerful pain relief: On the way to your brain, those pressure signals from your skin's nerve cells go through your spinal cord, one of your body's pain centers. And pressure signals travel faster than pain signals.

Your 12-Week Plan

I'm so proud of you for completing *The Woman's Guide to Strength Training: Dumbbells* program.

By dedicating yourself to it you've taken a significant step toward improving your strength.

Just because the program ended, doesn't mean your fitness journey does. Remember that consistency is key to lasting results. To maintain all of the strength you've gained, feel free to revisit stage three and try to challenge yourself with more workouts or by going up in weight slightly. By practicing the principles and techniques you learned in this program (reference page 16 for "4 Essential Elements of an Effective Strength-Training Routine"), you have the fundamental building blocks you need to continue working on having a strong, healthy body. Now's a great time to look back at your starting point from page 23. Do the exercises now feel easier? Can you do more reps? Celebrate how far you've come and continue to challenge yourself and work toward becoming the best version of YOU. Your journey to strength and empowerment is just beginning, and the best is yet to come!

Consider these self-reflection questions:

What were you surprised to learn about yourself during this program?

_____
_____
_____
_____

What changes have you experienced? List both the physical and mental.

_____
_____
_____
_____

How will you maintain the strength you gained?

_____
_____
_____
_____

Dumbbell Exercise Glossary

Upper Body

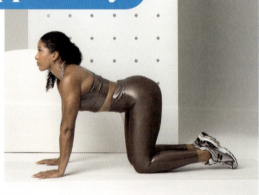
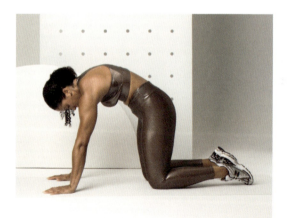

Cat Cow

MIND-MUSCLE CONNECTION FOCUS / Back and core

● Start on all fours with arms directly under shoulders and knees under hips, with spine in neutral alignment. ● Inhale and move into a "cow" pose by dropping belly toward mat and lifting chin and gaze toward ceiling as back arches. ● Exhale while shifting from "cow" past neutral to "cat" pose by drawing belly button into spine and rounding back. Keep neck relaxed and tilt head down. ● That's 1 rep.

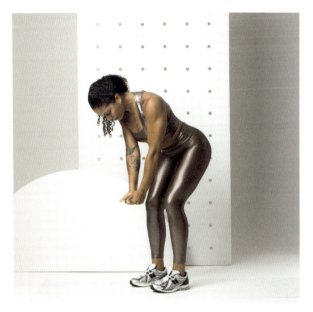
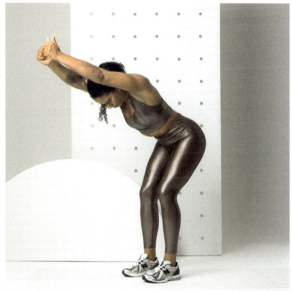
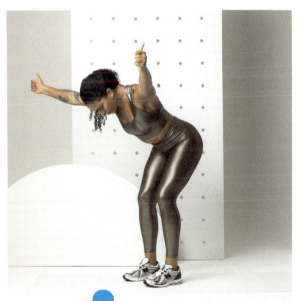
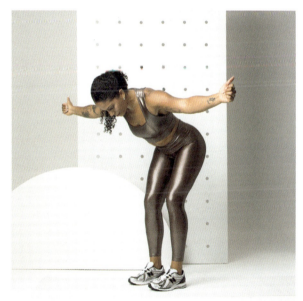

I-Y-T Raise
MIND-MUSCLE CONNECTION FOCUS / Back and rear deltoids

- Stand with feet shoulder-width apart and knees bent. Hinge forward at hips and let arms hang. - Raise arms overhead so body forms an I, then lower arms gradually so body forms a Y and then a T, holding for five seconds at each position. - That's 1 rep.

Dumbbell Exercise Glossary • Upper Body

Thread the Needle

MIND-MUSCLE CONNECTION FOCUS /
Shoulders, upper back, chest, and arms

- Start in a tabletop position with arms directly under shoulders and knees directly under hips.
- Lift right hand, arm straight towards the sky, then thread it under left shoulder so head can rest on floor facing left hand.
- Hold for 30 seconds. Imagine arm being gently pulled through to deepen stretch as upper back rotates.
- Repeat on left side.

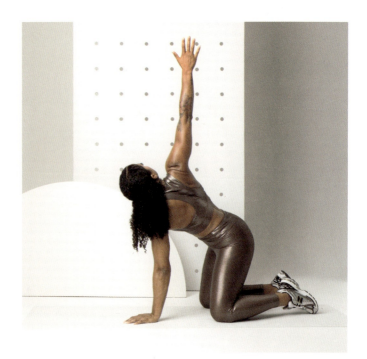

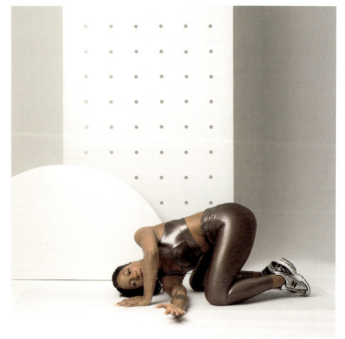

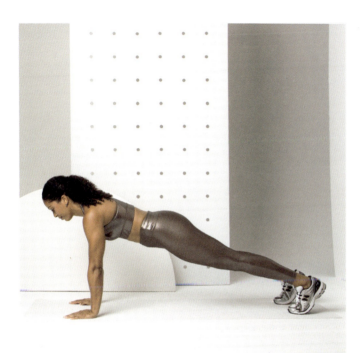

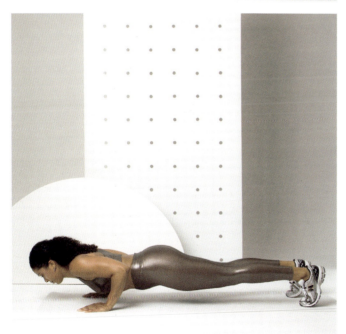

Pushup

MIND-MUSCLE CONNECTION FOCUS /
Arms, chest, back, and core

● Begin in high plank position, with feet a bit wider than hip-width apart, shoulders stacked over wrists, core engaged, and toes tucked. ● Body should form a straight line from shoulders to heels. Make sure neck is in-line with spine, shoulders are pulled back and away from ears, and glutes and quads are engaged. ● On an inhale, bend elbows to lower chest down toward floor, squeezing shoulder blades together and keeping core, quads, and glutes engaged. Upper arms should form 45-degree angles with sides. ● Once elbows are bent to 90 degrees or chest touches floor, exhale and push through hands to press body back up, maintaining engagement and that straight-line position. ● That's 1 rep.

Dumbbell Exercise Glossary • Upper Body

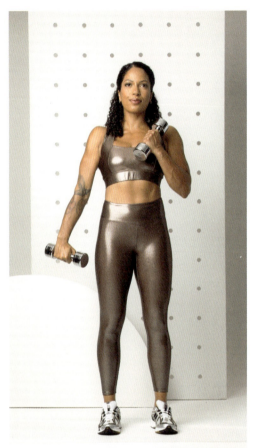 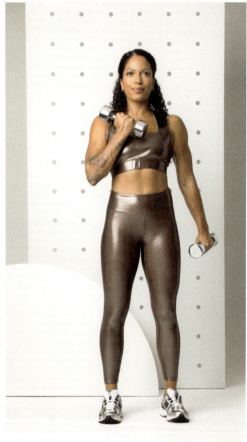

Cross-Body Alternating Biceps Curl

MIND-MUSCLE CONNECTION FOCUS / Biceps

- Stand with feet shoulder-width apart, with a dumbbell in each hand.
- Raise one dumbbell toward opposite shoulder. Return to start.
- Repeat on other side.
- That's 1 rep.

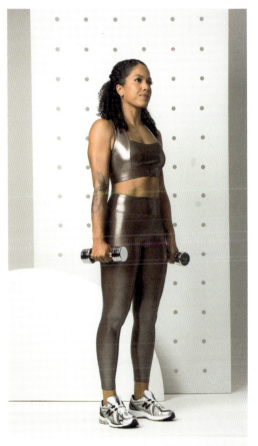
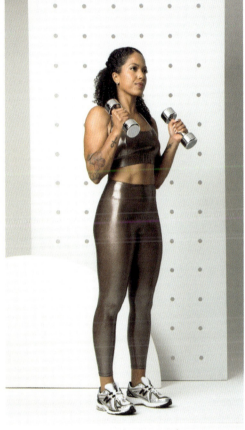

Hammer Curl

MIND-MUSCLE CONNECTION FOCUS / Biceps

● Stand with feet shoulder-width apart, a microbend in knees. ● Hold a pair of dumbbells at sides, palms facing toward sides of body, and keep back straight and chest up. Without moving upper arms, bend elbows and curl weights toward shoulders. ● Slowly lower weights back to starting position, straightening arms completely. ● That's 1 rep.

Dumbbell Exercise Glossary • Upper Body

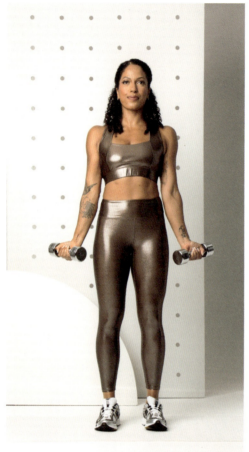
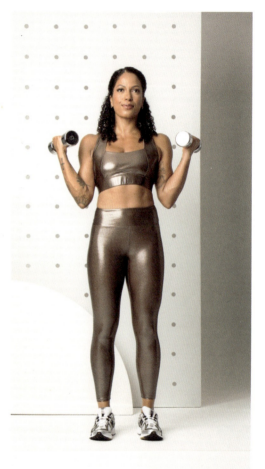

Wide Biceps Curl

MIND-MUSCLE CONNECTION FOCUS / Biceps

● Stand with feet shoulder-width apart, a microbend in knees. ● Hold a pair of dumbbells in each hand, forearms out at a 45-degree angle away from body. ● Without moving upper arms, bend elbows and curl weights toward shoulders. ● Slowly lower weights back to starting position, straightening arms completely. ● That's 1 rep.

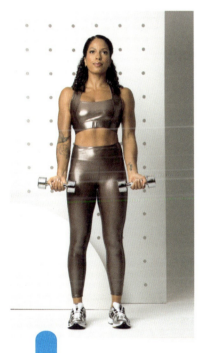
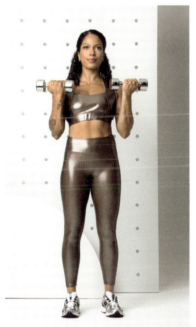
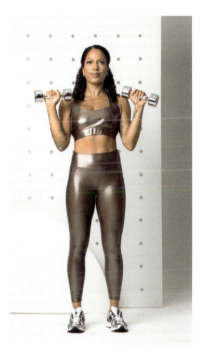

Zottman Curl

MIND-MUSCLE CONNECTION FOCUS / Biceps and forearms

● Stand with feet hip-width apart, holding weights in front of you, palms facing forward. ● Without moving upper arms, slowly curl weights toward shoulders. ● At top of curl, rotate wrists so palms face forward. ● Slowly lower them in that position. Rotate wrists and dumbbells back to starting position. ● That's 1 rep.

Dumbbell Exercise Glossary • Upper Body

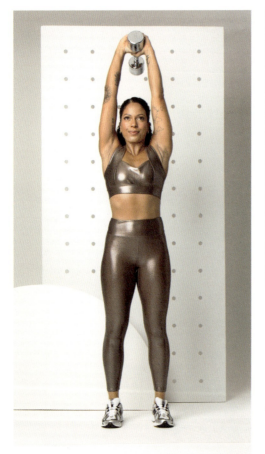
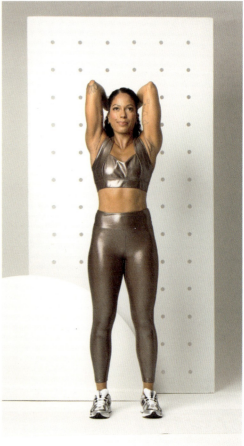

Overhead Triceps Extension

MIND-MUSCLE CONNECTION FOCUS / Triceps

• Start standing, gripping one dumbbell with both hands, and lift weight overhead, arms straight, feet hip-width apart. • Keeping upper arms by ears, bend elbows to lower weight slowly behind head and pause. • Straighten arms, returning to start. • That's 1 rep.

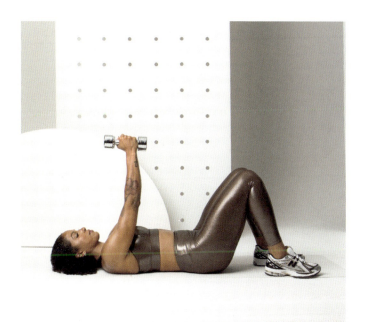

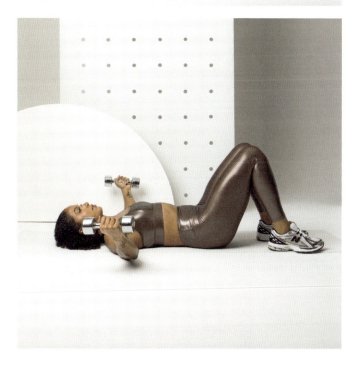

Chest Fly

MIND-MUSCLE CONNECTION
FOCUS / Chest

● Lie face up with knees bent and feet flat on floor. ● Grasp dumbbells with palms facing inward. ● Push dumbbells directly above your chest with lightly bent elbows, keeping wrists straight. ● Inhale and slowly lower dumbbells toward floor at shoulder height, maintaining a soft roundness with your arms (think: hugging a tree). ● Stop when back of upper arms touch mat. ● Exhale and slowly raise dumbbells back to the starting position while maintaining arc in your arms. ● That's 1 rep.

Dumbbell Exercise Glossary • Upper Body

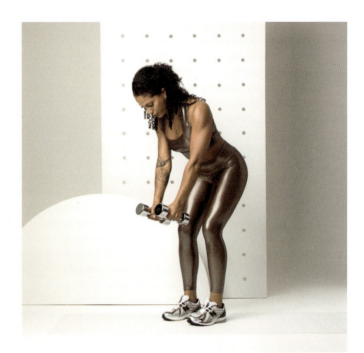

Reverse Fly

MIND-MUSCLE CONNECTION FOCUS / Rear deltoids

● Stand with feet hip-width apart, hips pushed back so torso is tilted forward 45 degrees and arms are extended straight down toward floor, hands holding weights, palms facing each other. ● Squeeze shoulder blades together and lift elbows wide to sides, then return to start. ● That's 1 rep.

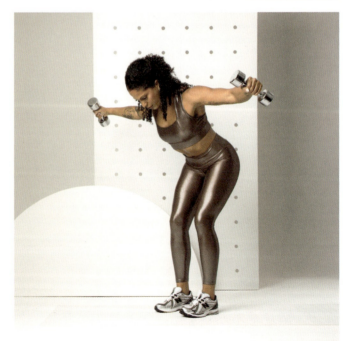

Alternating Reverse Fly
MIND-MUSCLE CONNECTION FOCUS / Rear deltoids

● Hold a pair of dumbbells and stand with feet hip-width apart and knees bent. ● Hinge forward at hips and let arms hang straight down from shoulders, palms facing body. ● Raise one arm out to side while squeezing shoulder blades together. ● Pause at top, then lower with control. ● Repeat on other side. ● That's 1 rep.

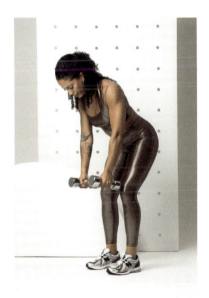
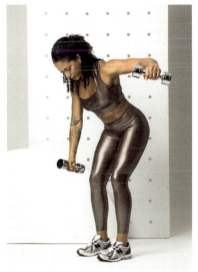
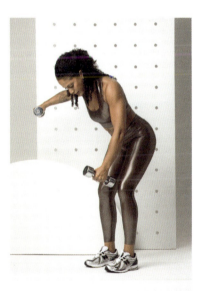

Dumbbell Exercise Glossary • Upper Body

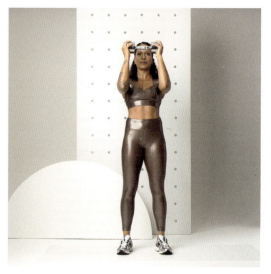
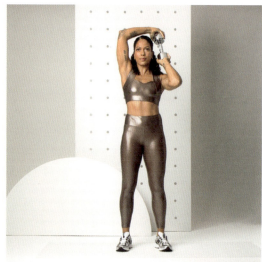
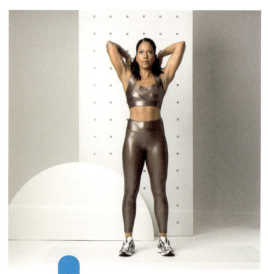
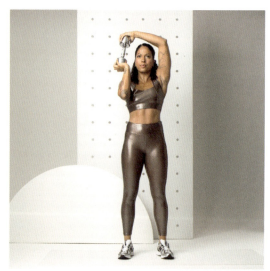

Halo

MIND-MUSCLE CONNECTION FOCUS / Shoulders, biceps, and core

● Start standing with feet hip-width apart holding ends of one dumbbell with both hands in front of face, elbows bent. ● Keeping both elbows bent, and rest of body still, slowly circle weight around head once, keeping it at eye level. ● That's 1 rep.

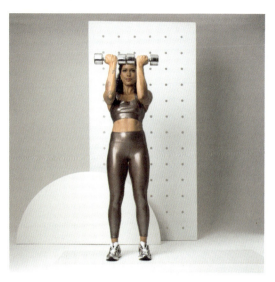
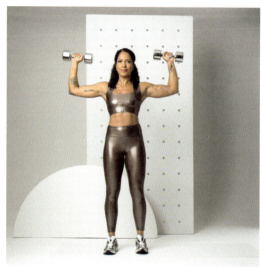

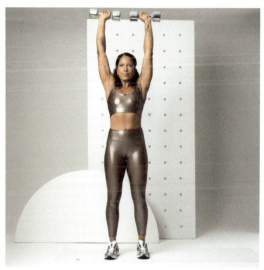

Arnold Press

MIND-MUSCLE CONNECTION FOCUS / **Shoulders and chest**

● Start standing with feet hip-width apart, holding a pair of dumbbells at shoulder height, with elbows bent and palms facing body. In one motion, bring elbows out wide to sides while rotating hands so palms face forward and pressing dumbbells overhead until arms are straight and biceps are by ears. ● Pause, then reverse movement to return to start. ● That's 1 rep.

Dumbbell Exercise Glossary • Upper Body

Bridge Chest Press

MIND-MUSCLE CONNECTION FOCUS / Chest, glutes, and core

- Lie face up on floor with knees bent and feet flat on floor.
- With a dumbbell in each hand, extend arms directly over shoulders, palms facing toward feet.
- Squeeze glutes to press hips off floor until torso forms a straight line.
- Squeeze shoulder blades together and slowly bend elbows, lowering weights out to the side, parallel with shoulders, until elbows form 90-degree angles.
- Slowly drive dumbbells back up to start, squeezing shoulder blades the entire time.
- That's 1 rep.

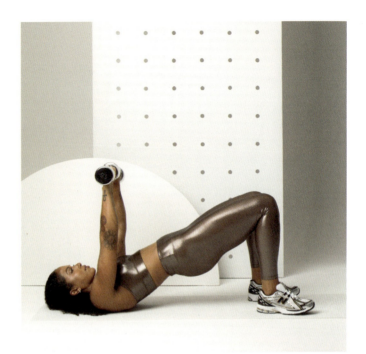

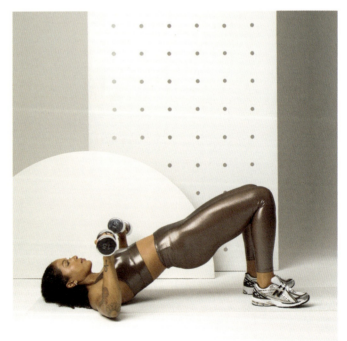

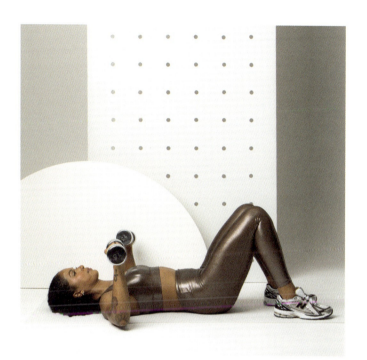

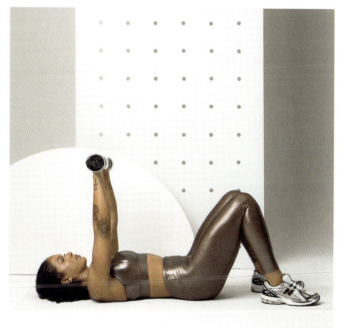

Chest Press

MIND-MUSCLE CONNECTION FOCUS / Chest

● Lie face up with knees bent and feet flat on floor. ● Holding a dumbbell in each hand, extend arms directly above shoulders, palms facing toes. ● Slowly bend elbows, lowering weights out to side until elbows form 90-degree angles. ● Drive dumbbells back up to starting position. ● That's 1 rep.

Dumbbell Exercise Glossary • Upper Body

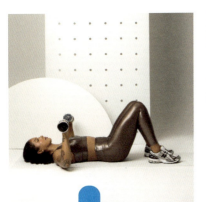 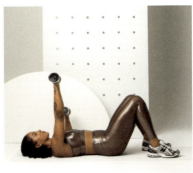 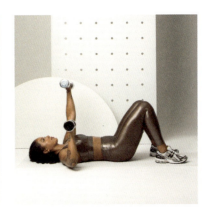

Alternating Chest Press

MIND-MUSCLE CONNECTION FOCUS / Chest

- Lie face up on floor with knees bent and feet planted flat on floor. • Hold a dumbbell in each hand and rest upper arms on floor with elbows bent at 90 degrees. • Upper arm should form a 45-degree angle with body. • Extend right arm up above shoulder. • Slowly bend right arm and lower it to side, until right elbow touches floor. • Repeat on left side. • That's 1 rep.

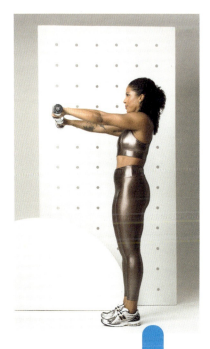 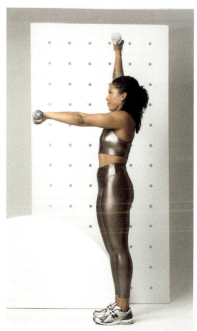 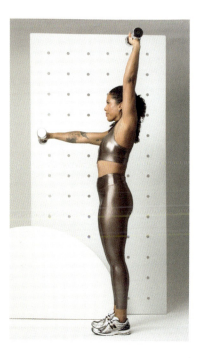

Gator Press

MIND-MUSCLE CONNECTION FOCUS / Shoulders

● Stand with feet hip-width apart, knees softly bent, and hold a dumbbell in each hand, arms raised in front of you at shoulder height, palms facing down. ● Keeping both arms straight, raise right arm overhead. ● Reverse to return to start; repeat on other side. ● That's 1 rep.

Dumbbell Exercise Glossary • Upper Body

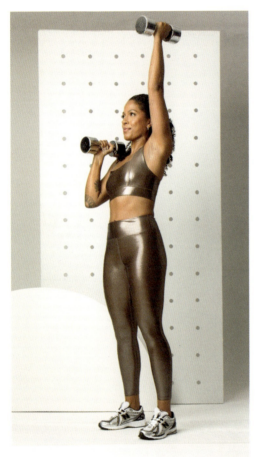
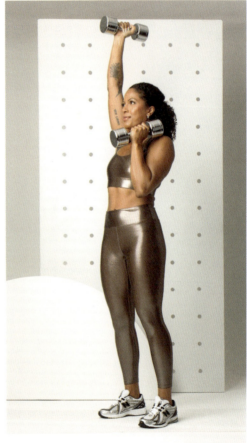

Dumbbell Seesaw Press

MIND-MUSCLE CONNECTION FOCUS / Shoulders

● Start standing with feet hip-width apart, holding dumbbells with left arm extended straight overhead, biceps by ear, and right arm bent, elbow narrow and weight at shoulder height. ● Switch arm positions so right arm presses straight up overhead and left is bent, then reverse simultaneously to return to start. ● That's 1 rep.

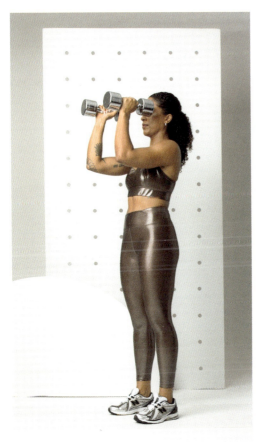
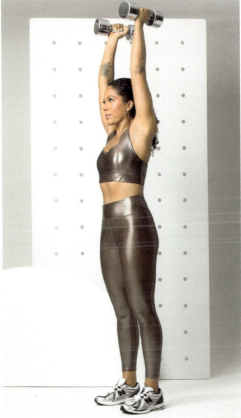

Shoulder Press

MIND-MUSCLE CONNECTION FOCUS / Shoulders

● Stand with feet hip-width apart, pelvis tucked and core engaged, holding dumbbells so head of weight is in front of eyes and elbows are bent 90 degrees. ● Press both hands overhead, without locking out elbows. ● Reverse movement to return to start. ● That's 1 rep.

Dumbbell Exercise Glossary • Upper Body

Kneeling Dumbbell Shoulder Press

MIND-MUSCLE CONNECTION FOCUS / Shoulders

- Kneel with knees under hips, holding dumbbells at shoulders, palms facing each other.
- Brace core and push weights directly overhead.
- Slowly lower dumbbells to return to start.
- That's 1 rep.

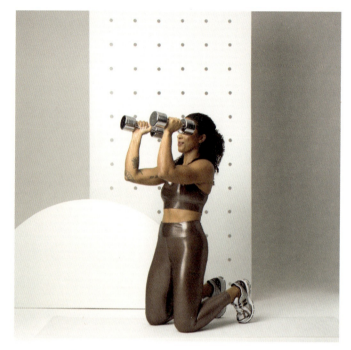

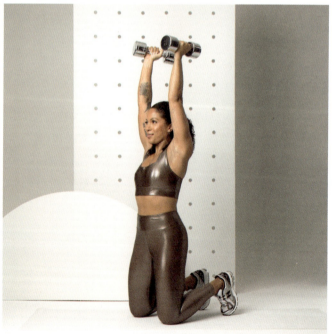

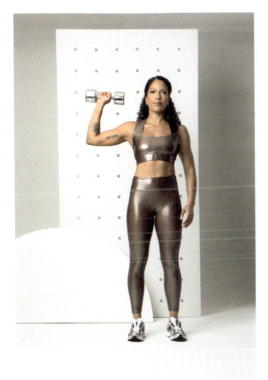
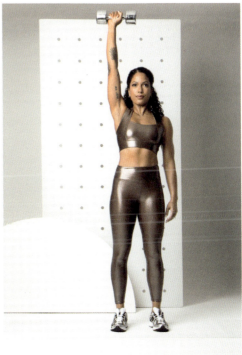

Single-Arm Shoulder Press

MIND-MUSCLE CONNECTION FOCUS / Shoulders and core

● Start standing with feet hip-width apart and holding a dumbbell in right hand at shoulder height. ● Engage glutes and press arm with weight overhead until elbow is straight and biceps is next to ear. ● Lower arm with control. ● That's 1 rep.

Dumbbell Exercise Glossary • Upper Body

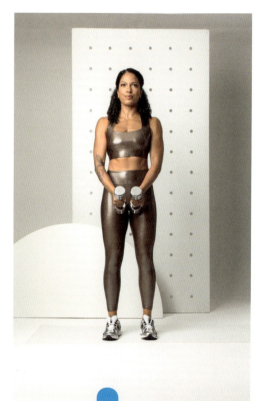 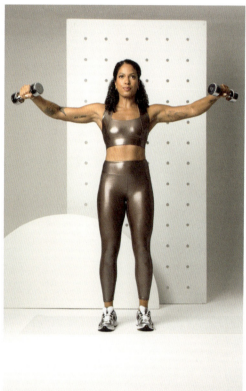

Lateral Raise

MIND-MUSCLE CONNECTION FOCUS / Shoulders

● Stand with feet hip-width apart and arms in front of thighs holding dumbbells. ● Allowing a gentle bend in elbows, lift arms out to sides until parallel to floor. ● Keep palms facing down throughout. ● Slowly reverse motion to lower arms to sides. ● That's 1 rep.

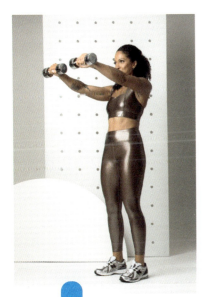
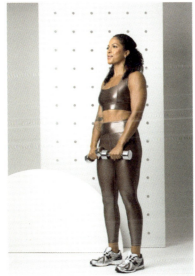
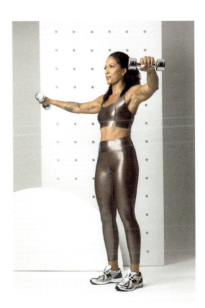

Alternating Front and Lateral Raise

MIND-MUSCLE CONNECTION FOCUS / Shoulders

● Stand with knees slightly bent, feet hip-width apart, and arms down by sides, holding dumbbells in each hand. ● Raise arms in front until hands reach shoulder height. ● Lower arms with control to sides. ● Raise arms out wide until parallel to floor. ● Lower arms slowly to return to start. ● That's 1 rep.

Dumbbell Exercise Glossary • Upper Body

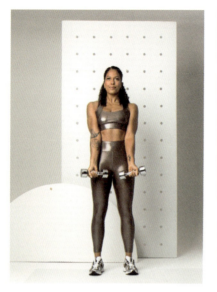
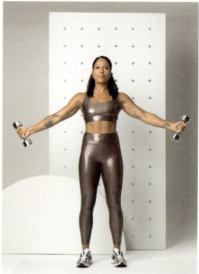
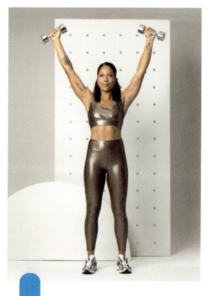
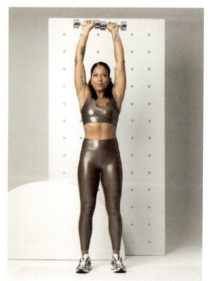

Dumbbell Rainbow

MIND-MUSCLE CONNECTION FOCUS / Shoulders and biceps

● Stand with feet hip-width apart, knees slightly bent, and hold a dumbbell in each hand at thighs, palms facing up. ● With a slight bend in elbows, slowly lift weights out to sides, then up to touch above head. ● Reverse to return to start. ● That's 1 rep.

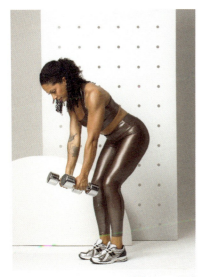 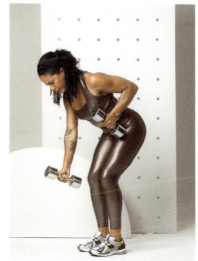 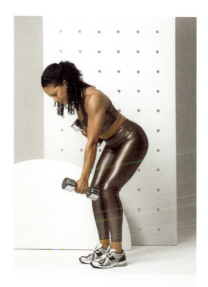

Alternating Bent-Over Row
MIND-MUSCLE CONNECTION FOCUS / Back

● Start with feet hip-width apart, holding one dumbbell in each hand with palms facing each other. ● Hinge at hips, keeping head in line with tailbone. ● Bracing core, pull left elbow back until left wrist is near ribs. ● Lower with control to return to start position. ● Repeat on right side. ● Lower with control to return to start. ● That's 1 rep.

Dumbbell Exercise Glossary • Upper Body

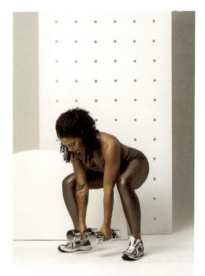 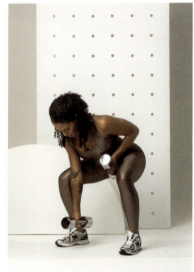 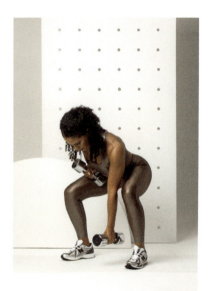

Gorilla Row

MIND-MUSCLE CONNECTION FOCUS / Latissimus dorsi

- Stand with feet wider than hip-width apart, toes pointed slightly out. - With a flat back, hinge forward at hips to grip dumbbells on floor. - Bend and pull left elbow back and up until just above back, while other dumbbell hovers above floor. - Lower arm with control to reverse movement until weight hovers above floor.
- Then repeat on right side. - That's 1 rep.

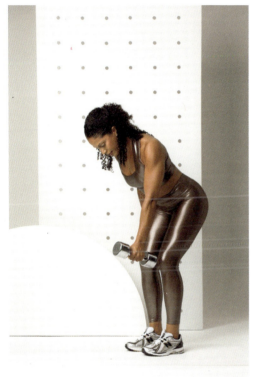
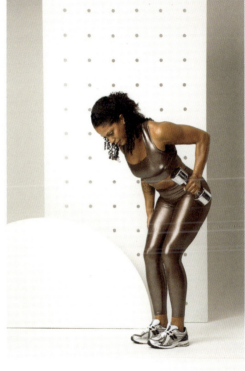

Dumbbell Single-Arm Row

MIND-MUSCLE CONNECTION FOCUS / Latissimus dorsi

● Stand with feet hip-width apart, holding dumbbell in left hand; hinge forward, knees slightly bent and weight hanging at arm's length. ● Keeping core tight, squeeze shoulder blades toward spine to pull weight to chest. ● Pause, then slowly lower back to start. ● That's 1 rep.

Dumbbell Exercise Glossary • Upper Body

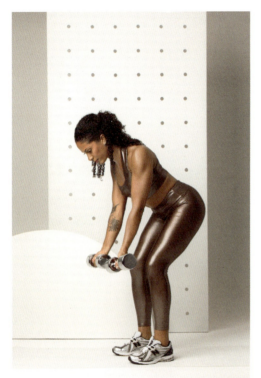 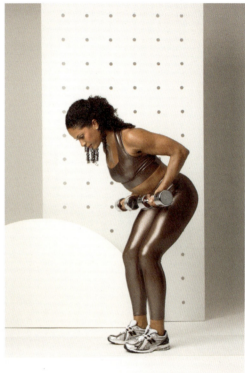

Underhand Bent-Over Row

MIND-MUSCLE CONNECTION FOCUS / Biceps

● Grasp a pair of dumbbells with an underhand grip and stand with feet hip-width apart, knees slightly bent. ● Bend forward from hips until back is almost parallel to floor, arms hanging directly from shoulders and palms facing away from body. ● Brace core, then pull weights toward rib cage, squeezing shoulder blades together. ● Pause, then lower to return to start. ● That's 1 rep.

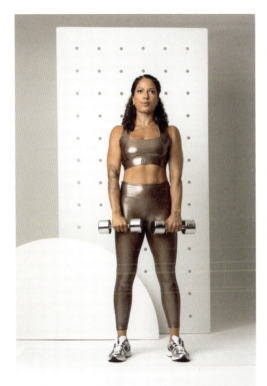
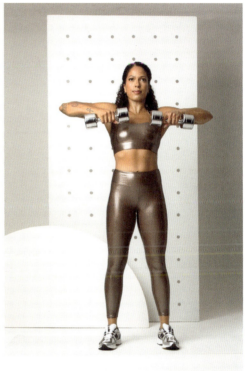

Upright Row

MIND-MUSCLE CONNECTION FOCUS / Shoulders and upper back

● Stand with feet hip-width apart, arms reaching toward floor, with hands holding weights against thighs and palms facing body. ● Pull elbows wide and up to slightly above shoulders, so hands reach chest height, then return to start. ● That's 1 rep.

Dumbbell Exercise Glossary • Upper Body

Skull Crusher

MIND-MUSCLE CONNECTION FOCUS / Triceps

- Lie on back with knees bent and feet planted on floor.
- Hold a dumbbell in each hand and extend arms straight above chest.
- Without moving upper arms, bend at elbows to lower dumbbells toward sides of head.
- Extend dumbbells back to ceiling.
- That's 1 rep.

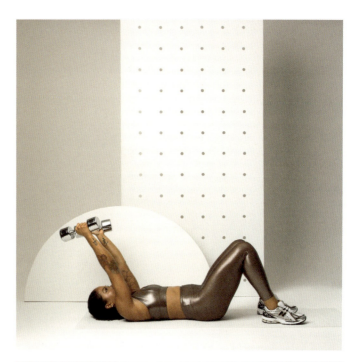

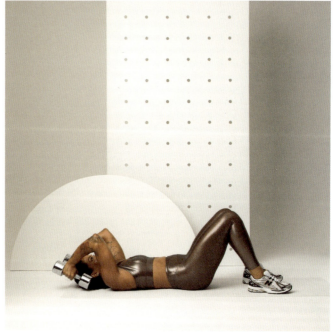

Core

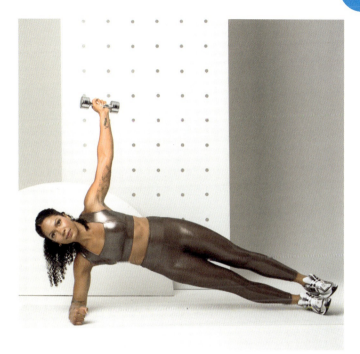

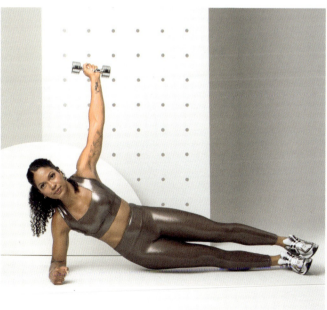

Side Plank Hip Dip

MIND-MUSCLE CONNECTION FOCUS / Core

● Start in a side plank on right forearm with left arm extended toward ceiling, holding a dumbbell. ● Use obliques to lower hips toward mat with control. ● Reverse movement to return to start. ● That's 1 rep.

Dumbbell Exercise Glossary • Core

Deadbug

MIND-MUSCLE CONNECTION FOCUS / Core and hip flexors

● Lie on back with arms extended over chest and legs bent 90 degrees (knees above hips). ● Keep lower back pressed to floor, brace core, then slowly and simultaneously extend and lower right leg until heel nearly touches floor and extend and lower left arm until hand nearly touches floor overhead. ● Pause, then return to start; that's 1 rep.

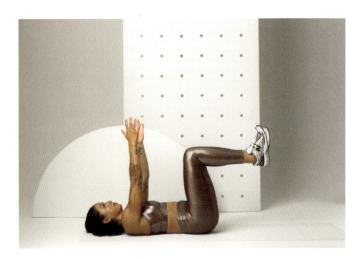

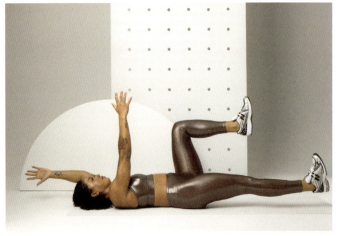

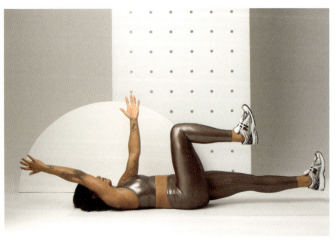

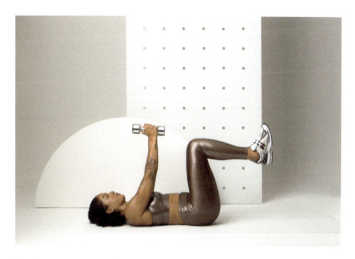
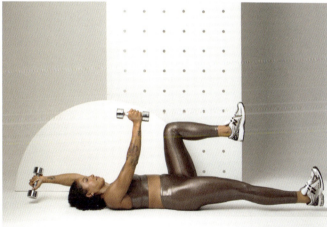
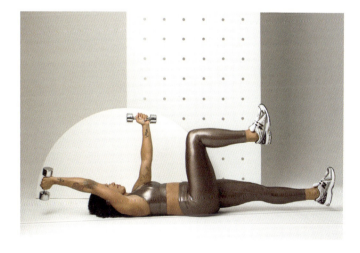

Loaded Deadbug

MIND-MUSCLE CONNECTION FOCUS / Core and hip flexors

● Lie face up on floor with knees and hips bent 90 degrees, arms extended over shoulders, a light dumbbell in each hand. ● Keeping core and glutes tight, slowly extend right leg and lower toward floor while bringing left arm overhead. ● Return to start; that's 1 rep. ● Repeat on other side and continue alternating.

Dumbbell Exercise Glossary • Core

Russian Twist

MIND-MUSCLE CONNECTION FOCUS / Core

- Sit on floor with hands clasped in front of chest and lean upper body back until abs are engaged. Feet may remain on the ground or lift slightly off to enhance difficulty.
- Rotate torso to right side so that right elbow is hovering just off mat.
- Keep lower body still while rotating upper body to left side until left elbow is just off mat.
- Return to center.
- Gaze follows hands as you move.
- That's 1 rep.

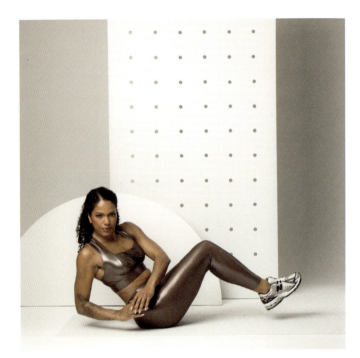

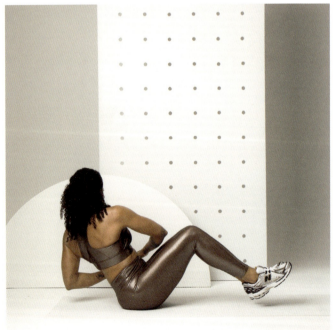

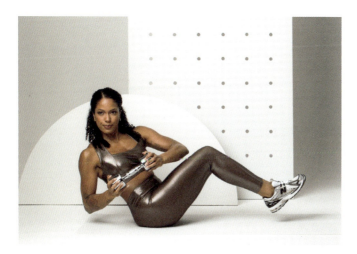

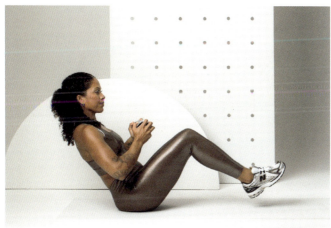

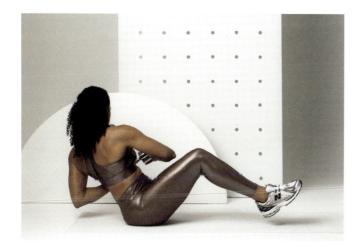

Weighted Russian Twist

MIND-MUSCLE CONNECTION FOCUS / Core

● Sit on floor holding a dumbbell in front of chest and lean upper body back until abs are engaged. ● Feet may remain on the ground or lift slightly off to enhance difficulty. ● Rotate torso to right side so that right elbow is hovering just off mat. ● Keep lower body still while rotating upper body to left side until left elbow is just off mat. ● Return to center. ● Gaze follows hands as you move. ● That's 1 rep.

Dumbbell Exercise Glossary • Core

Toe Touch

MIND-MUSCLE CONNECTION FOCUS / Core

- Lie face up, holding one dumbbell in both hands and extending arms and legs to ceiling.
- Lift head and shoulder blades off floor as you reach dumbbell toward toes.
- Keep lower back glued to floor and arms and legs stretched toward ceiling throughout rep.
- With control, lower head and shoulders back to floor.
- That's 1 rep.

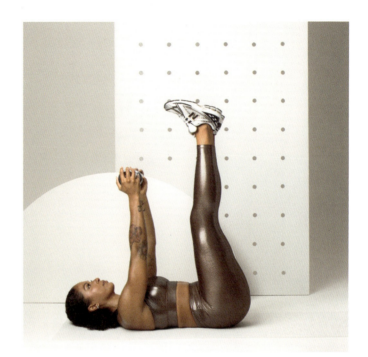

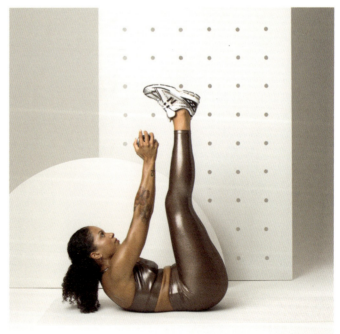

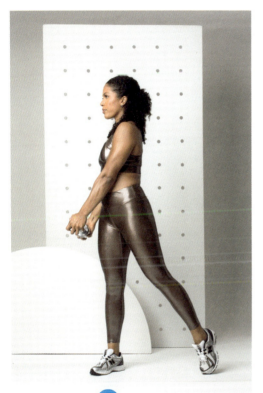
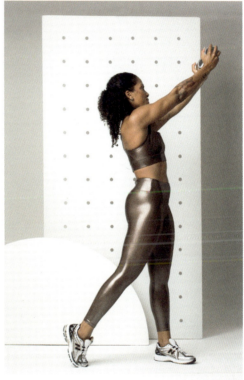

Wood Chop

MIND-MUSCLE CONNECTION FOCUS / Core and shoulders

● Stand with feet wider than hip-width apart and hold a dumbbell with both hands, bend knees, and bring weight outside right hip. ● Keeping arms straight, rotate torso and shoulders to bring weight across body, finishing over left side. ● Return to start. ● That's 1 rep.

Dumbbell Exercise Glossary • Lower Body

Lower Body

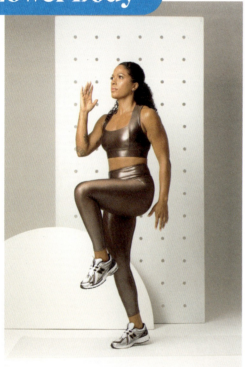
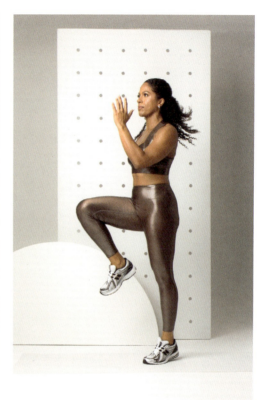

High Knee

MIND-MUSCLE CONNECTION FOCUS / Core and legs

- Start standing. ● Run in place, driving knees toward chest. ● Use arms and try to go as fast as you can. ● Complete as recommended.

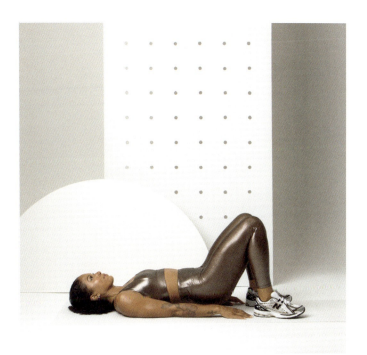

Glute Bridge

MIND-MUSCLE CONNECTION FOCUS / Glutes

- Lie face up with knees bent and feet flat on floor.
- Squeeze glutes and lift hips off floor until body forms a straight line from knees to shoulders.
- Pause at top, then lower back down to starting position.
- That's 1 rep.

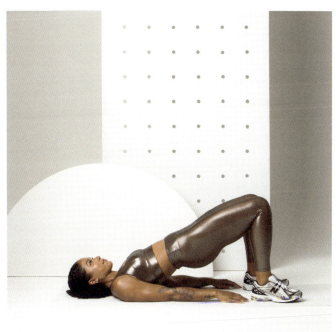

Dumbbell Exercise Glossary • Lower Body

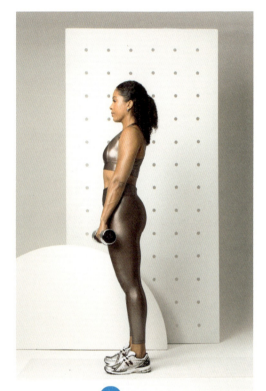
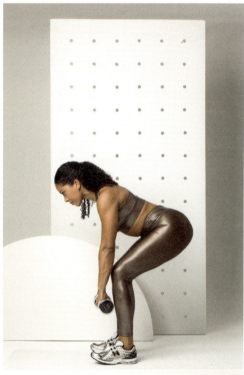

Romanian Deadlift

MIND-MUSCLE CONNECTION FOCUS / Glutes and hamstrings

- Stand with feet hip-width apart, holding dumbbells close to body by hips, palms facing toward body. ● Keeping spine long, send hips back with control as you hinge forward at waist. ● Keeping dumbbells close to body, lower weights to shins, or as far down as you can without curving spine. ● Pause, then reverse movement to return to start, engaging glutes and core at top. ● That's 1 rep.

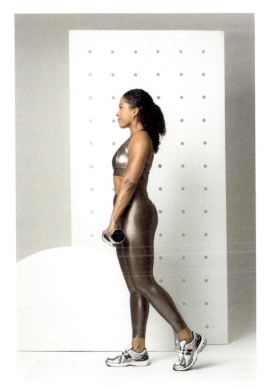
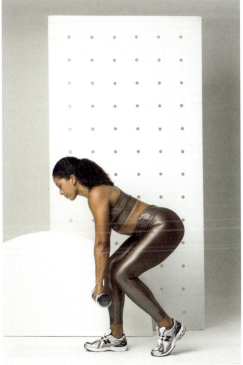

Staggered-Stance Deadlift

MIND-MUSCLE CONNECTION FOCUS / Glutes and hamstrings

● Stand with feet hip-width apart, then move left foot back so toes are slightly behind right heel (most of your weight should be on right foot). ● Keeping spine long, send hips back as you hinge at waist. ● Lower weights to shin, or as far as you can without curving spine. ● Pause, then reverse, engaging glutes and core at top. ● That's 1 rep.

Dumbbell Exercise Glossary • Lower Body

Weighted Hip Thrust

MIND-MUSCLE CONNECTION FOCUS / Glutes

- Lie face up with knees bent and feet flat on floor.
- Place dumbbell on lap and grip both ends.
- Drive hips up toward ceiling so shoulders, hips, and knees form a straight line. Squeeze glutes at top.
- Pause for a moment at top, keeping core braced.
- Then, in a slow and controlled motion, lower hips back toward floor.
- That's 1 rep.

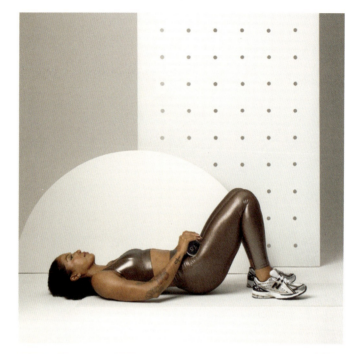

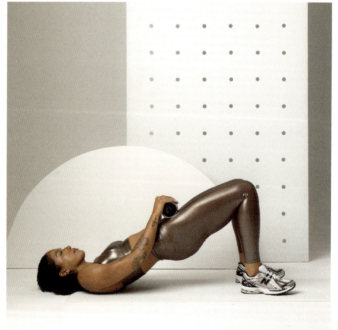

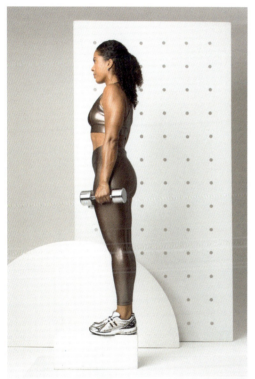 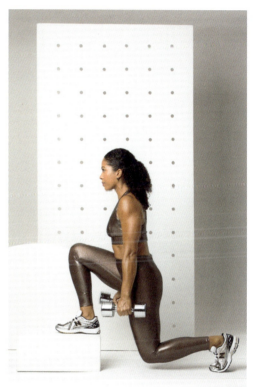

Deficit Reverse Lunge

MIND-MUSCLE CONNECTION FOCUS / Glutes and hamstrings

● Stand on a six-inch step or box and hold a pair of dumbbells at sides at arm's length. ● Keeping torso tall, step backward off box with left leg and slowly lower body until right knee is bent at least 90 degrees and left knee nearly touches floor. ● Push through right heel to return to start. ● That's 1 rep.

Dumbbell Exercise Glossary • Lower Body

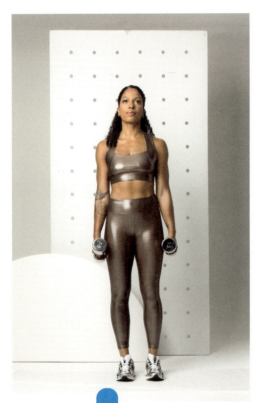
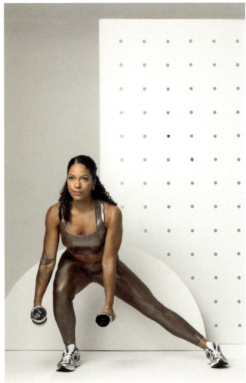

Lateral Lunge

MIND-MUSCLE CONNECTION FOCUS / Glutes, hamstrings, and quads

- Start with feet shoulder-width apart, toes pointed straight forward.
- Step out with right foot as wide as possible.
- Engage through right heel as hips drop down and back while keeping left leg straight, and keeping both soles of feet on floor and toes pointed straight forward.
- Make sure right knee is tracking over right foot the whole motion.
- Powerfully "punch" right heel into floor to push back to full standing start position.
- That's 1 rep.

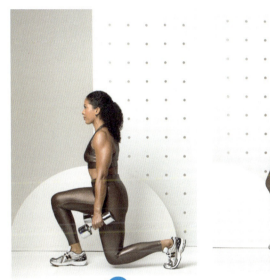
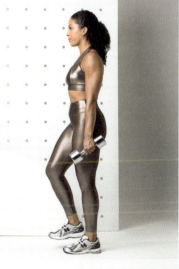
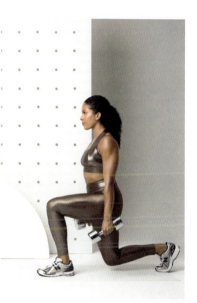

Two-Way Lunge

MIND-MUSCLE CONNECTION FOCUS / Glutes, hamstrings, and quads

● Holding a dumbbell in each hand, step right foot forward and bend knees until front leg is nearly parallel to floor. ● Press through right heel to stand; immediately step right foot back and bend knees to lower into reverse lunge. ● Return to start. ● That's 1 rep.

Dumbbell Exercise Glossary • Lower Body

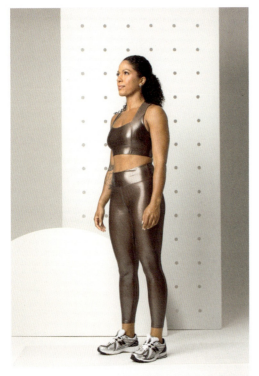 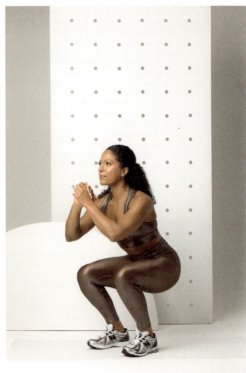

Squat

MIND-MUSCLE CONNECTION FOCUS / Glutes, hamstrings, and quads

● Start standing with feet hip-width apart, toes pointed out slightly. ● Keeping head in line with tailbone, shift hips back and bend at knees. ● Lower down until thighs are parallel with floor. ● Drive up through heels to return to standing. ● That's 1 rep.

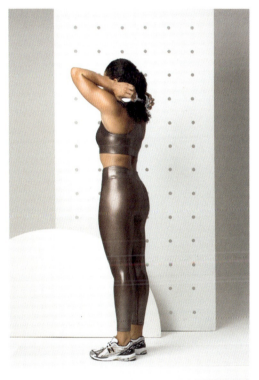
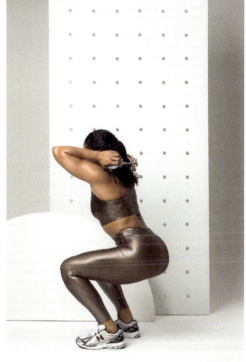

Back Squat

MIND-MUSCLE CONNECTION FOCUS / Glutes, hamstrings, and quads

● Start standing with feet parallel and shoulder-width apart, holding a dumbbell in both hands and resting behind neck. ● Engage core, push hips back, and lower down slowly until thighs are parallel with floor. ● Press through feet to reverse movement and return to start. ● That's 1 rep.

Dumbbell Exercise Glossary • Lower Body

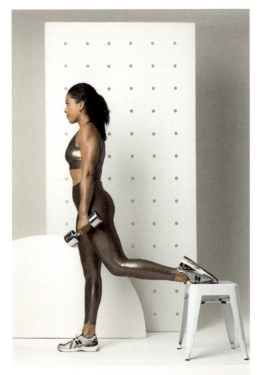
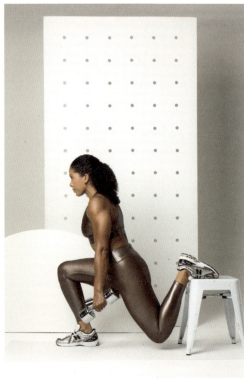

Bulgarian Split Squat

MIND-MUSCLE CONNECTION FOCUS / Glutes

- Start standing tall with right foot forward and left back, top of left foot resting on a box, holding a dumbbell in each hand. ● Shift weight into front right foot, engage core, keep torso upright, and bend at both knees to lower body until right thigh is parallel with the floor.
- Press through right foot to straighten legs and return to start position. ● That's 1 rep.

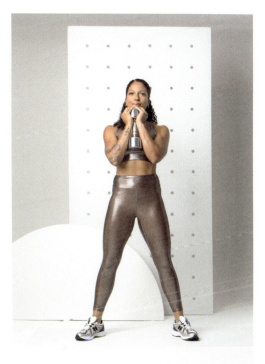
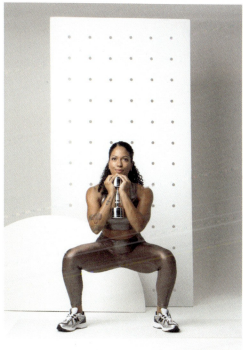

Goblet Squat

MIND-MUSCLE CONNECTION FOCUS / Core, quads, and glutes

- Stand with feet slightly wider than hip-width apart, holding one dumbbell vertically in both hands at chest height. ● Elbows should be close to rib cage. ● Bend knees and lower hips into a squat, keeping chest upright. ● Pause, then drive through heels and glutes to stand.
- That's 1 rep.

Dumbbell Exercise Glossary • Lower Body

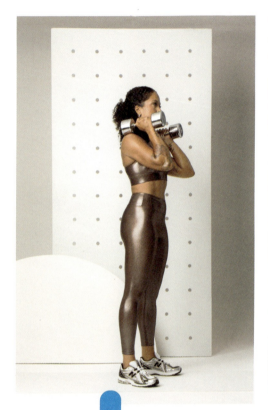
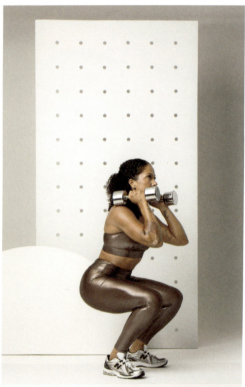

Front Racked Squat

MIND-MUSCLE CONNECTION FOCUS / Quads, glutes, and hamstrings

● Stand with feet hip-width or slightly wider apart and hold two dumbbells at shoulders with elbows slightly raised and toes pointed forward or slightly out. ● Maintain an engaged core and breathe in through nose while lowering hips in a sitting motion, keeping chest upright. ● Build tension through body during descent, moving weight into heels. (Avoiding losing tension at bottom of lift.) ● Push through floor with inner and outer soles of feet to return to standing, breathing out through mouth and tensing glutes and quads. (Body should feel tight and compact throughout movement.) ● That's 1 rep.

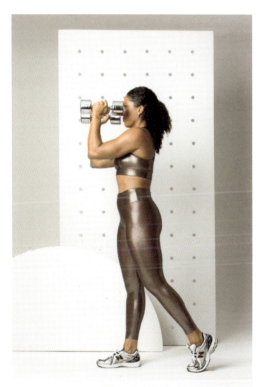
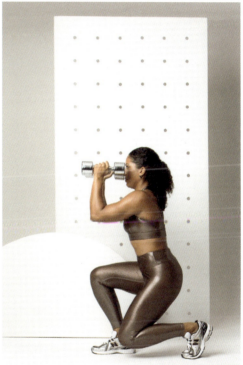

Staggered-Stance Front Racked Squat

MIND-MUSCLE CONNECTION FOCUS / Glutes and hamstrings

● Stand with feet hip-width apart, holding two dumbbells racked at eye level. ● Take a step back with left foot so it acts as a kickstand. ● Bend knees and lower hips into a squat keeping chest upright and weight in right foot. ● Drive through front heel and glutes to stand. ● That's 1 rep

Dumbbell Exercise Glossary • Lower Body

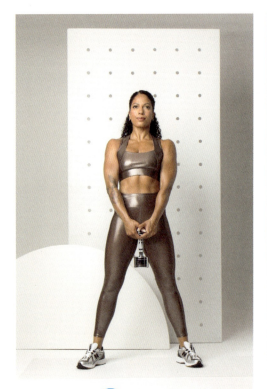
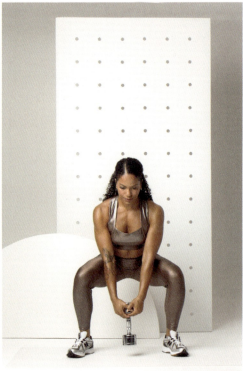

Dumbbell Sumo Squat

MIND-MUSCLE CONNECTION FOCUS / Glutes

● Start standing with feet wider than hip-width apart, toes pointed out at 45 degrees, torso slightly forward, holding a dumbbell with both hands in front of you. ● Inhale, bend knees, and sink hips down until thighs are parallel to floor. Make sure to drive knees outward. ● Exhale and drive through heels to return to starting position. ● That's 1 rep.

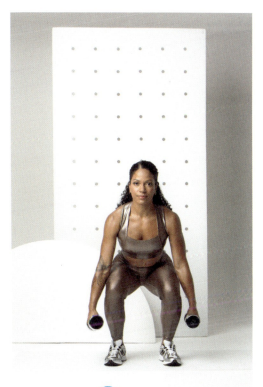
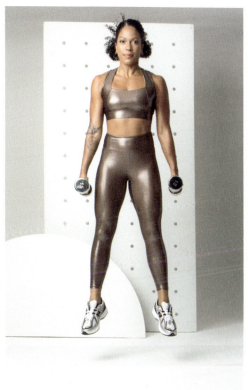

Squat Jump

MIND-MUSCLE CONNECTION FOCUS / Quads and hamstrings

● Stand with feet shoulder-width apart and hold a pair of dumbbells, arms by sides. ● Sit back into a squat until thighs are nearly parallel to floor, then press through heels to straighten legs and jump off floor; immediately lower into next rep. ● That's 1 rep.

Dumbbell Exercise Glossary • Lower Body

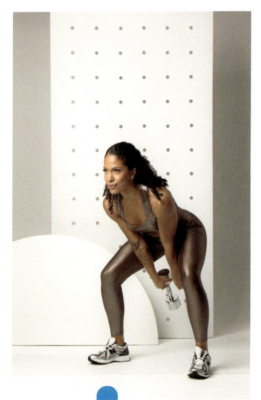
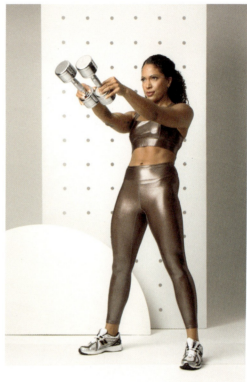

Dumbbell Swing

MIND-MUSCLE CONNECTION FOCUS / Glutes and hamstrings

- Stand with feet shoulder-width apart, toes pointed slightly out.
- Hold a dumbbell by the end in each hand.
- Keeping spine straight, hinge forward at waist and bend knees to bring dumbbells between legs.
- Powering movement with glutes, hips, and hamstrings (not arms), stand and swing dumbbells up to chest height.
- Reverse move to return to start, letting dumbbells swing back with control.
- That's 1 rep.

Total Body

World's Greatest Stretch

MIND-MUSCLE CONNECTION FOCUS / Quads, hamstrings, and back

- Start in a high plank position with a flat back and wrists under shoulders.
- Step left foot forward and plant it outside of left hand to achieve a deep lunge position.
- Right knee can be straight or slightly bent resting down on mat.
- Lift left hand from mat, bend left elbow, and reach left forearm down toward mat between left foot and right hand.
- Hold position for a second. Rotate trunk toward left and reach left hand toward ceiling.
- Hold this position for a second.
- That's 1 rep.
- Perform required reps, return to starting position, then repeat on opposite side.

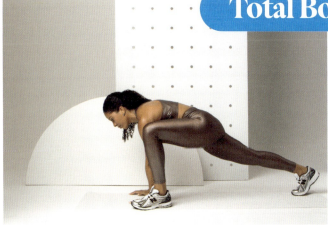

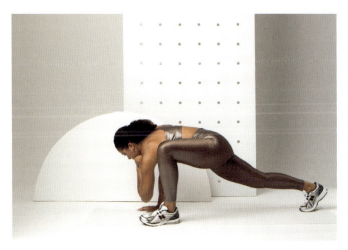

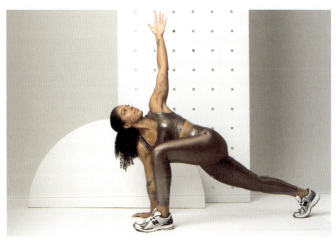

Dumbbell Exercise Glossary • Total Body

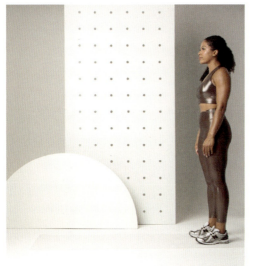
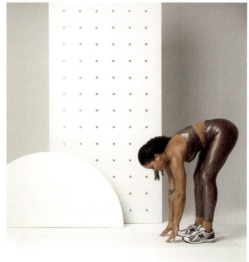
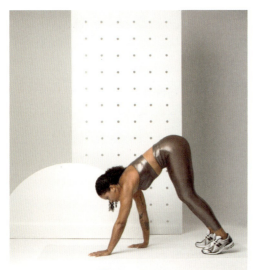
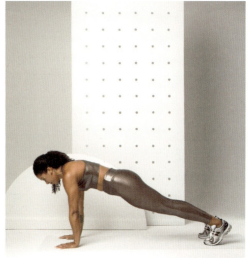

Plank Walkout

MIND-MUSCLE CONNECTION FOCUS / Core and arms

- Begin standing at back of mat with feet under hips and hands at sides. ● Fold forward at waist and bring palms to floor, then begin walking hands forward, stopping in a high plank position with wrists under shoulders and legs extended straight. ● Reverse movement to return to start. ● That's 1 rep.

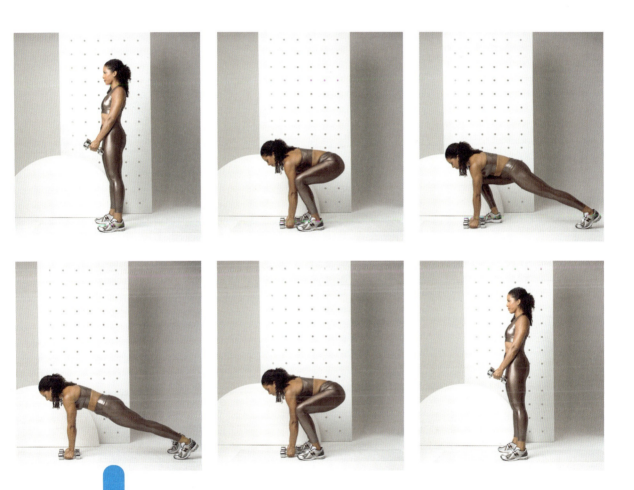

Modified Burpee

MIND-MUSCLE CONNECTION FOCUS / Hamstrings and core

● Stand with feet slightly wider than hip-width apart, holding a dumbbell in each hand against thighs, palms facing each other. ● Squat and place dumbbells on floor between feet. ● Keeping hands on dumbbells, walk back into a plank position and hold. ● Reverse movement by walking back into squat, then stand. ● That's 1 rep.

Dumbbell Exercise Glossary • Total Body

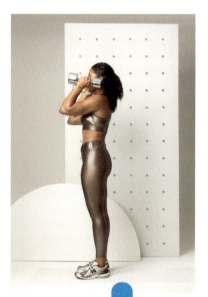
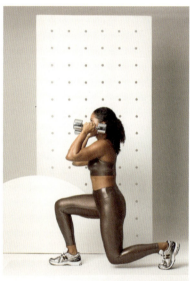
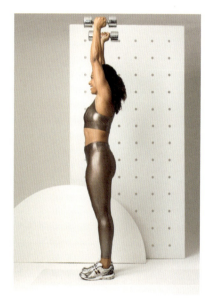

Reverse Lunge to Press

MIND-MUSCLE CONNECTION FOCUS / Shoulders, core, and hamstrings

- Hold a pair of dumbbells at shoulder height, palms facing in, feet about hip-width apart. • Step left foot back and bend knees until right thigh is parallel to floor. • In one smooth motion, push through right heel to stand while pressing weights directly above shoulders until arms are fully extended. • That's 1 rep. • Lower weights to shoulders while stepping right foot back to start next rep; continue alternating sides.

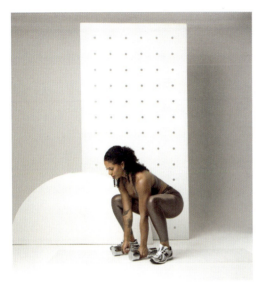
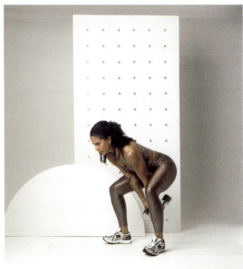
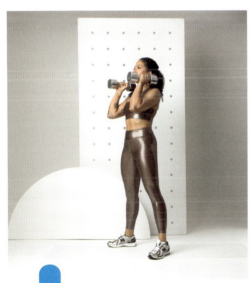
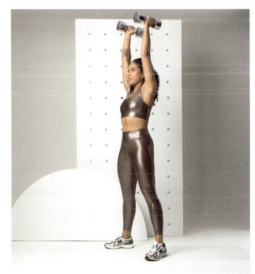

Modified Devil Press

MIND-MUSCLE CONNECTION FOCUS / Glutes, core, and shoulders

● Squat low with feet shoulder-width apart, holding dumbbells directly below shoulders and resting on floor to start. ● Hinge at hips and swing both dumbbells between legs. ● Once weights are behind you, contract glutes and thrust hips forward. ● Raise dumbbells to shoulders, palms facing each other and elbows narrow as you stand upright. ● Bend knees slightly, then power through legs to press dumbbells straight up overhead until arms are extended. ● Lower dumbbells to floor to return to start. ● That's 1 rep.

Dumbbell Exercise Glossary • Total Body

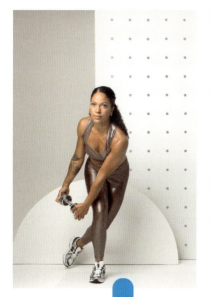 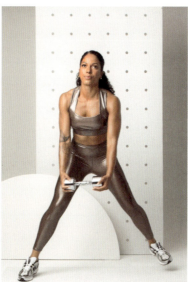 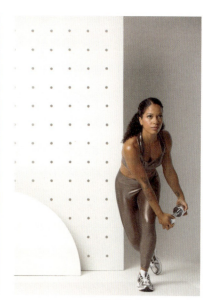

Dumbbell Speed Skater

MIND-MUSCLE CONNECTION FOCUS / Quads and core

- Hold both ends of a dumbbell, jump to right, and as you land, cross left leg behind you, bend knees, and lower weight outside of right leg.
- Quickly hop back and repeat on other side. • That's 1 rep.

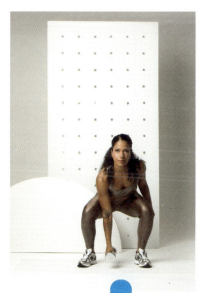 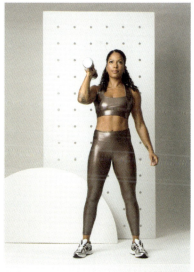 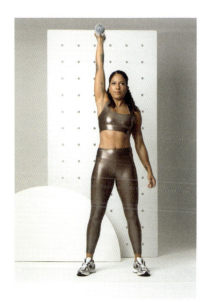

Squat and Snatch

MIND-MUSCLE CONNECTION FOCUS / Hamstrings and shoulders

- Start in a squat with a dumbbell between feet, holding it in one hand with an overhand grip. ● Power through hips, knees, and ankles to stand and accelerate dumbbell upward. ● Shrug shoulders and engage core to "flip" dumbbell, engaging lower body to support weight. ● Using lower body and core, extend dumbbell overhead with power. ● Reverse move to return to start. ● That's 1 rep.

Dumbbell Exercise Glossary • Total Body

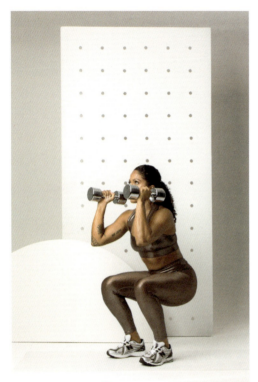 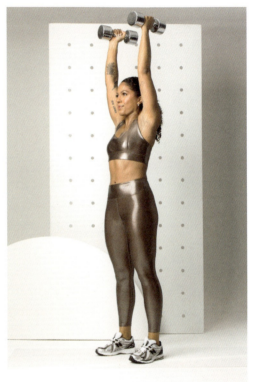

Squat Thruster

MIND-MUSCLE CONNECTION FOCUS / Glutes, shoulders, and hamstrings

● Stand with feet slightly wider than shoulder-width apart and toes turned slightly out. ● Hold a dumbbell in each hand at shoulder height, palms facing each other. ● Bend knees and sit back until thighs are parallel to floor. ● Push pelvis forward as you stand and extend arms, pressing weights overhead. ● Slowly reverse movement to immediately lower into next rep. ● That's 1 rep.

Notes:

Notes:

Notes:

NOTES

Notes:

Notes:

This book is intended as a reference volume only, not as a medical manual. The information given here is designed to help you make informed decisions about your health. It is not intended as a substitute for any treatment that may have been prescribed by your doctor. If you suspect that you have a medical problem, we urge you to seek competent medical help.

© 2024 by Hearst Magazines, Inc.

All rights reserved. No part of this publication may be reproduced or transmitted in any form or by any means, electronic or mechanical, including photocopying, recording, or any other information storage and retrieval system, without the written permission of the publisher.

Women's Health® is a registered trademark of Hearst Magazines, Inc.

Photography by Eli Schmidt

Styling by Rose Lauture (Heroine Sport bra and leggings: cover; Gigi C romper, Mejuri hoops: 11, 39, 73; Heroine Sport bomber, bra, and shorts; Machete hoops: 12, 47, 93; Reebok sports bra and leggings; APL sneakers; Machete hoops: 14, 24, 55, 113; Alo Yoga bra; The Upside shorts; Nike sneakers; Mejuri earrings: 19, 31, 133; Heroine Sport bra and leggings; New Balance sneakers; Mejuri earrings: 32-37, 40-44, 48-52, 56-60, 64-70, 74-80, 84-90, 94-100, 104-110, 114-130, 134-206)

Hair and Makeup by Paige Achkov

Book design by Hanna Varady

Library of Congress Cataloging-in-Publication Data is on file with the publisher.

ISBN 978-1-955710-38-1

Printed in China

2 4 6 8 10 9 7 5 3 1 hardcover

HEARST

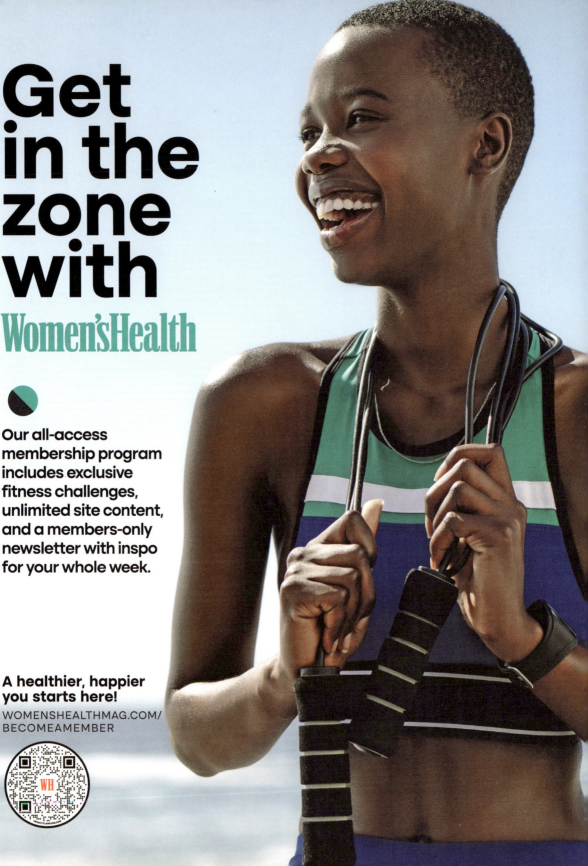

Get in the zone with

Women'sHealth

Our all-access membership program includes exclusive fitness challenges, unlimited site content, and a members-only newsletter with inspo for your whole week.

A healthier, happier you starts here!
WOMENSHEALTHMAG.COM/
BECOMEAMEMBER